P9-ANY-055

Science Library

Biology of Menopause

The Causes and Consequences of Ovarian Ageing

Biology of Menopause

The Causes and Consequences of Ovarian Ageing

R. G. Gosden

Department of Physiology
University Medical School
Edinburgh, Scotland

1985

ACADEMIC PRESS

(Harcourt Brace Jovanovich, Publishers)

London   Orlando   San Diego   New York
Toronto   Montreal   Sydney   Tokyo

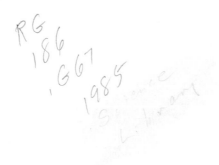

COPYRIGHT © 1985, BY ACADEMIC PRESS INC. (LONDON) LTD.
ALL RIGHTS RESERVED.
NO PART OF THIS PUBLICATION MAY BE REPRODUCED OR
TRANSMITTED IN ANY FORM OR BY ANY MEANS, ELECTRONIC
OR MECHANICAL, INCLUDING PHOTOCOPY, RECORDING, OR
ANY INFORMATION STORAGE AND RETRIEVAL SYSTEM, WITHOUT
PERMISSION IN WRITING FROM THE PUBLISHER.

ACADEMIC PRESS INC. (LONDON) LTD.
24–28 Oval Road
LONDON NW1 7DX

United States Edition published by
ACADEMIC PRESS, INC.
Orlando, Florida 32887

British Library Cataloguing in Publication Data

Gosden, R. G.
    Biology of menopause: the causes and consequences
    of ovarian ageing.
    1. Menopause
    I. Title
    612'.665   RG186

Library of Congress Cataloging in Publication Data

Gosden, R. G.
    Biology of menopause.

    Bibliography: p.
    Includes index.
    1. Menopause. I. Title. [DNLM: 1. Menopause.
WP 580 G676b]
RG186.G67   1985   612'.665   84-14516
ISBN 0–12–291850–9 (alk. paper)

PRINTED IN THE UNITED STATES OF AMERICA

85 86 87 88   9 8 7 6 5 4 3 2 1

To Mother and Carole

Foreword

The impressive expansion of life expectancy which has occurred this century in most developed countries has been accompanied by a large increase in the number of elderly women. Although the average woman will spend over one-third of her life after the menopause, we know very little about the factors which determine the onset of ovarian failure. Ignorance in this area reflects our lack of knowledge of the process of growth, development and degeneration of follicles. In this monograph, Roger Gosden has placed in biological context the events surrounding the continued ageing of the reproductive system, including the ovaries, of which the last menstrual period is an obvious landmark.

The oocytes are amongst the longest surviving cells in the body. A finite number of oocytes are formed in fetal life, and when they are exhausted ovarian failure occurs. With this prolonged period of storage it is hardly surprising, therefore, that the incidence of congenital abnormalities due to chromosome abnormalities rises with maternal age. Cumulative exposure to radiation and other potential mutagenic agents increases the risk of errors in meiosis occurring. The normal functioning of the ovary as an endocrine gland is totally dependent on an adequate supply of healthy gametes. Hence, as the ovary ages a variety of abnormalities in its function, as indicated by a disturbance in the pattern of menstruation, become common. The experimental models in laboratory rodents which are available for the study of these observations are discussed with authority by Roger Gosden, who has made a life study of ovarian failure.

The social significance of the menopause varies greatly from one culture to the next. In Hindu India and certain parts of northern Nigeria the appearance of the first grandchild marks the end of the second "ashrama", or period of procreation, after which sexual activity should cease. The menopausal grandmother acquires a different, more prestigious, place in society and may be permitted to take a more active part in decision making. In Western society the menopause usually coincides with marked changes in personal circumstances, e.g. children leaving home, and is regarded by many as a depressing reinforcement of the ageing process. The decline in production of ovarian steroids, including oestradiol, results in short-term symptoms and long-term changes in the reproductive and skeletal system. It is against the biological consequences of ageing that the risks and benefits of oestrogen replacement therapy must be viewed. This book is a timely summary of our present knowledge in this important area.

David T. Baird
Professor of Obstetrics
and Gynaecology
University of Edinburgh

Preface

There should be good reasons for adding to the current flood of scientific literature, especially since the task of writing a monograph is a long and lonely one. This book was written for research workers, clinicians and students who have a special interest in the biology of the ageing reproductive system, of which the human menopause is a central issue. It deals with the causes of ovarian failure in mid-life, the associated physiological and behavioural changes and the preceding decline in fecundity and fertility. Despite widespread interest in this subject, no one until now has attempted to tackle the subject as a whole. A number of books have been written for the non-scientific reader who is concerned about "menopausal problems", but the professional scientist and clinician are faced with a widely dispersed literature. I felt that there was still time for an author with sufficient temerity to bring together the many aspects of reproductive system ageing and show the extent to which these are interrelated.

This book is primarily concerned with human biology, but in some sections where direct evidence is lacking there are detailed accounts of animal research, and often this is interesting in its own right. By way of introduction to some of the chapters, I have outlined historical concepts leading to our present knowledge of the physiology and biochemistry of reproduction. This is intended to help readers who are not well acquainted with the subject to appreciate the less tractable problems of ageing. However, to maintain balance and economy, it has been necessary to be highly selective. Originally, I planned to shun all practical issues in reproductive medicine, but, as the book evolved, the provinces of the biologist and clinician seemed less distinct, and some mention of contraception and hormone replacement therapy became desirable. Nevertheless, these topics have been tackled primarily from the scientific standpoint, and I leave questions of clinical management of subfertility and postmenopause to others having appropriate experience and expertise. Discussion of the psychological changes of middle age, apart from those of a sexual nature or connected with ovarian ageing, are beyond the scope of this book, and as the title plainly indicates my subject is strictly the female of the species. Males are not exempt from ageing of their sexual functions, but a term other than "menopause" is needed for their less discrete changes. A good deal more research needs to be done before as detailed a story can be written about them.

Acknowledgements

Had I not received so much encouragement and support I might never have begun this volume, never mind completed it. My thanks are due first to Bob Edwards for launching me into a research field which has held my interest over the years and now forms the basis of this work. Helpful advice and criticism during the evolution of the final manuscript were given by several colleagues, namely, David Baird, Terry Baker, Tony Bramley, Ann Chandley, Tuck Finch, Don McLaren, Evelyn Telfer; and I appreciate guidance given by the editorial staff at Academic Press Inc. (London) Ltd. at all stages of the project. Nevertheless, I accept full responsibility for the more speculative hypotheses which are proposed or endorsed here. It is a pleasure to record unstinting support and service from librarians in the Erskine Medical Library, the Centre for Reproductive Biology and elsewhere in the university. Authors and publishers have kindly granted permission to reprint data; their contributions are specifically acknowledged in the accompanying tables and legends. Much of the illustrated material was prepared with the help of the Medical Illustration Unit of Edinburgh University, with many figures being drawn by the medical artist, Ian Lennox. Finally, I thank my wife, Carole, for patience and encouragement throughout the project and for important contributions at every stage: searching the literature, providing literary criticism and proofreading; and if there is any humanity in the way I have presented the science, it is mainly due to her influence.

April 1984

R.G.G.
University Medical School
Edinburgh, Scotland

Contents

Biology of Menopause

The Causes and Consequences of Ovarian Ageing

1

Distribution of Menopause

1.1. Introduction

The reproductive system changes in appearance and function more obviously than any other system during maturation and ageing. Indeed, the human female lifespan can be divided into three phases according to menstrual activity, the first and last menses (menarche and menopause) marking the transitions. These two milestones of life are merely expressions of underlying continuous changes; they signify the attainment of hormonal thresholds determining the initiation and maintenance of ovarian cycles. These changes affect aspects of reproduction besides menstruation and may be expressed as variations in fertility during menstrual life.

The pattern of rising and waning reproductive potential is not peculiar to our species, but can be seen in other animals in conditions of captivity or domestication. It is not, however, a universal pattern in vertebrates, amongst which some remarkable life cycles have emerged. For example, the bluehead wrasse (*Thalassoma bifasciatum*) changes sex during ageing, and both sexes of marsupial mice (*Antechinus* sp.) have a single burst of intensive reproductive activity which is quickly followed by sterility, senescence and death (Diamond, 1982).

According to the evolutionary paradigm, every life cycle, no matter how bizarre, must confer special advantages for reproduction of the species. Can, then, the menopause and the long postcyclic phase of life in man be of adaptive value? This is doubtful. Of course, the crucial facts of hominid evolution are lacking, but we can be fairly sure that early ovarian deterioration was not selected since evolutionary fitness can be maximized only among young, reproductively active individuals. Although postreproductive individuals no longer contribute directly to the gene pool of the next generation, it has been suggested that some benefits may accrue indirectly; they can expend energy in caring for offspring of their kin, thus increasing the survivorship of their line (Mayer, 1982). Quite apart from the difficulties of obtaining credible evidence for this hypothesis, it would appear that any benefits are far outweighed by the costs of menopause, namely, the increased morbidity and mortality of the offspring and mother during the declining years of fertile life. There are several indications that women are not physiologically well adapted to the postmenopause, further countering the argument that it has an evolutionary advantage.

Human menopause is probably a novelty, although its potential has existed for a long time because germ cells are continuously depleted from a non-renewable store. The potential for ovarian failure also exists in animals today. According to this viewpoint, menopause is an artefact of human civilization which emerged when our growing mastery of the environment increased our survivorship.

Our understanding of the origins of life patterns is bound to colour our attitudes to the menopause. It is, however, much more hazardous to draw firm conclusions in this area than on the surer ground of the physiology and biochemistry of menopause which form the basis of this book.

1.2. Terminology

The term ''menopause'', which was introduced in the nineteenth century, means the time when menstrual cyclicity ceases irreversibly. It is popularly used to describe a vague period near the close of menstrual life, but in scientific and medical parlance it simply designates the last menses. This is usually, though not universally, identified retrospectively after 12 months of amenorrhoea. Often it is tacitly assumed that the underlying cause of menopause is primary and permanent ovarian failure. This distinguishes it from the loss of menses after hysterectomy, in which occult ovarian cycles may continue, and from seasonal ovarian involution in some animals, which is reversible. Postmenopausal vaginal bleeding is, of course, a continuing possibility, but extraovarian factors are usually responsible.

Wilbush (1979) states that it was de Gardanne (1816) who coined the term ''la ménespausie'' to replace the more cumbersome description ''cessation des ménstrues''. This was shortened in the second edition of his book to ''ménopause''. This term was soon absorbed into the English language because of its precision in expressing the essentially feminine nature of the condition. The tendency to use this word to describe gonadal atrophy in ageing men ought to be resisted.

Various prefixes have been added to describe the phases surrounding or involving menopause, but there are no generally agreed-on definitions of them. In this book the definitions recommended by the World Health Organization (1981) have been adopted. They are illustrated in Fig. 1.1 and defined as follows.

Menopause: Permanent cessation of menstruation resulting from loss of ovarian follicular activity.

Perimenopause: This term is used synonymously with the word ''climacteric'' (L. *klimakter:* rung of a ladder). It indicates a variable period spanning a

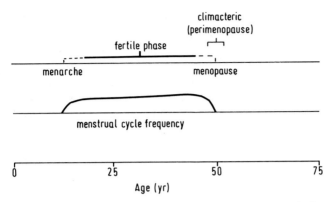

Fig. 1.1. Schematic diagram illustrating definitions and timing of events in the reproductive life-span of women.

few years on either side of the menopause when characteristic symptoms and signs of ovarian involution are present.

Postmenopause: The entire span of life following the last menses.

Premenopause: This is an unsatisfactory term because it can imply any period preceding the menopause, although many authors restrict its meaning to a short but poorly defined period before the climacteric.

1.3. Historical Recognition

The statistical probability of surviving to the age of menopause was relatively low until spectacular developments occurred in public health and medicine earlier this century. However, sufficient numbers of women have survived to this age for writers even in the distant past to remark about the phenomenon of menopause. When the author of Genesis stated that "it ceased to be with Sarah after the manner of women", he indicated the familiarity of this natural event. Many other documents from ancient Greece and Rome and from medieval Europe confirm this knowledge, although we cannot rely on them for accurate information on the exact age of menopause in those times (Amundsen and Diers, 1970, 1973; Post, 1971).

In the past, the loss of menstrual activity was widely believed to be directly responsible for the physical and psychological distress of the climacteric. The catamenial flow was thought to be a route for eliminating "peccant matter and morbid humour, sometimes acrimonious and malignant, whose retention never fails to be extremely injurious . . . to the constitution" (Fothergill, 1776). This concept of the role of menstruation was responsible for the stigma of impurity and the rituals attached to this stage of the cycle in some societies. Treatment of symptoms was carried out by "sage femmes" and "granny women" during recent centuries in Western Europe and was designed to counteract the retention of menses (menochesis) and thereby eliminate the accumulated "poisons". Such treatments involved traditional emmenagogues, but if these were unsuccessful, the excretion of retained "poisons" was promoted at alternative sites: through the skin and/or gut by purgatives, enemata, sinapisms, moxas, cupping or leeches or, finally, by the methods of the barber surgeons—phlebotomies or various "issues" (Wilbush, 1979).

These procedures were practised regularly as a means of increasing the attractiveness of women of high status. However, according to exhaustive studies of the historical literature by Wilbush (1979), menopausal symptoms or complaints were not recorded until the time of social upheavals in post-Revolutionary France. This period was remarkable for the growth of medical and paramedical French literature dealing with women, and especially with climacteric symptoms. Wilbush suggested that these symptoms are modified by social and historical conditions, a conclusion that is endorsed by recent cross-cultural surveys described in the next section.

During the nineteenth century, the time-honoured notions of the role of menstruation and the significance of menopause underwent revolutionary changes as a result of increasing scientific attention. The discovery of the effects of electricity on the body by Galvani (1737–1798) and others led to the conclusion that a wide variety of disorders might have an electrical basis. Georg Prochaska (1749–1820), a Viennese physiologist, proposed a neural mechanism for controlling the gonads, and thus, the effects of castration and the symptoms of the menopause were thought to be nervous reflexes or "ganglionic" disorders (e.g. Tilt, 1857).

Although the significance of autonomic factors in climacteric symptoms is accepted, the early views have been modified by the major endocrinological paradigm of our time. The evidence proving that the ovary is an organ of internal secretion was collated in an important work published by F. H. A. Marshall (1910). In subsequent decades the major task of isolating and chemically identifying the ovarian steroids was carried out, being substantially completed by the mid-1930s. This knowledge provided the basis for a new evaluation of the significance of menopause and its biological consequences.

Public interest in the menopause has increased in recent times because it has become popular for women to consult medical practitioners about climacteric symptoms. The profession can now offer an effective hormonal remedy, albeit a controversial one (Chapter 7). Interest has been heightened by a remarkable change in the age structure of developed countries during the past century. This change is illustrated by census data and projections for Scotland (Fig. 1.2), and similar trends are found elsewhere. The number of women of postmenopausal

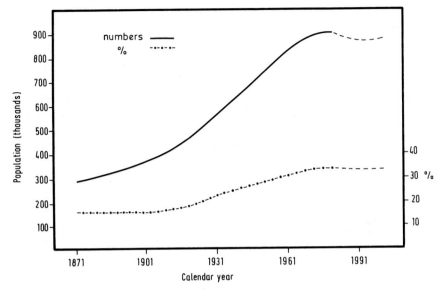

Fig. 1.2.   Number and percentage of women aged 50 years and older in Scotland from 1871 and projected forward until 2001. (From Government Actuary's Department, Registrar General for Scotland.)

age (i.e. age >49 years) has increased threefold since 1871, and as a fraction of the total population they have doubled to reach one-third. The reasons for this demographic shift are complex, involving interactions between fertility, age-specific mortality and migration. The present pattern is mainly attributed to high fertility in the past and a significant improvement of survival rates (Gray, 1976). In Scotland, life expectancy at birth increased from 43.5 to 74.4 years between 1871 and 1977 (i.e. 71%), whereas that at age 50 rose from 21 to 27.5 years (31%). Therefore, increased survival of children to middle age has had a greater impact on the size of the postmenopausal population than lower mortality rates in old age. Demographic forecasts are usually hazardous, but it is widely assumed that the size of the postmenopausal population will be stable during the next 2 decades unless there are radical and unexpected changes in mortality rates amongst the elderly. Consequently, the special problems of biological ageing, including menopause, will continue to be major forces in defining health care priorities into the next century.

1.4. Symptomatology

It is necessary to make some comment about the symptoms (i.e. subjective aspects) of the climacteric even though their biological significance is clouded by associated social and psychological factors of middle age. In some societies, particularly in the West, where youth and beauty are emphasized, the menopause can be a social stigma, and it often coincides with domestic or professional crises in the family. In other societies (e.g. in Rajasthan, amongst some Indian women of high caste) the menopause is associated with an increase in social standing which approaches, but does not quite reach, that of men (van Keep and Humphrey, 1976; Ware, 1979). It is not, therefore, surprising that attitudes towards menopause and the frequency with which symptoms are reported vary in different cultural settings. Some general patterns have emerged from the many surveys of climacteric symptoms, and they can be illustrated by comparative studies of ethnic groups within the same country.

In an Israeli study of five distinct ethnic groups (Jews of central European, Persian, Turkish and North African origin, and one Arab group), substantially different attitudes to menopause were found even though the range of somatic complaints was similar (Maoz et al., 1977). Hot flushes (flashes) and sweating were the predominant symptoms. Persian women experienced the greatest degree of discomfort, and Europeans suffered the least. Arab women were the most positive in their attitudes to menopause and Persians the least positive. Although higher income and education are associated with fewer or less intense symptoms during climacteric years (Jaszmann et al., 1969a; van Keep and Humphrey, 1976), the explanation of the Israeli data is undoubtedly more complex than this. The authors pointed out that there is no simple dichotomy of symptoms according to social background (traditional versus modern) and emphasize the possible effects of the relationship with the spouse and his attitudes. In another cross-cultural study, significant differences were found between Cuban and Jewish women in the United States (Flint and Garcia, 1979). Cubans expressed more negative attitudes to menopause and, perhaps as a consequence, experienced more symptoms than Jews. The following factors may be important in determining individual and ethnic differences in climacteric symptoms: (1) the social significance of menstruation and the escape from the stigma of menstruation that follows menopause in some cultures, (2) the social significance of childlessness, (3) the social status of postmenopausal women, (4) attitudes of husbands towards their postmenopausal wives, (5) the level of socio-economic deprivation experienced at the time, (6) the degree of change in the role of women at this time and the availability of new or alternative roles and (7) the availability of medical help for perimenopausal problems (World Health Organization, 1981).

A large number of symptoms are associated with the climacteric, and they are similar in character whether menopause is spontaneous or induced. Several observers have reported that they are of greater intensity when menopause is precocious or follows ovariectomy (oophorectomy) (e.g. Chakravarti et al., 1977). It is difficult to distinguish symptoms specific to menopause from those that are due to other ageing processes or social factors. This distinction is, of course, imperative for those involved in management of climacteric problems. Symptoms can be divided into two groups according to whether they involve genital tissue. Some of them have an obvious, direct causal relationship to the altered endocrine environment (e.g. irregular menstruation, dyspareunia), whereas others are related indirectly and have an autonomic basis (e.g. vasomotor disorders, perspiration, palpitations). Some psychogenic disturbances may be secondary to these symptoms (e.g. insomnia, loss of sex drive), but the aetiology of others is less obvious and probably more complex (headaches, irritability, depression, dizziness). There are, in addition, other consequences of menopause which are not immediately apparent but develop insidiously during the postmenopausal years (osteoporosis, atheromatosis).

Since most though not all women experience climacteric symptoms (80–85%) (Medical Women's Federation, 1933) and since similar symptoms are reported in cross-cultural studies, some of them evidently have a biological basis. The most common symptom is the hot flush, which is associated with another autonomic disorder, namely, inappropriate sweating (Thompson *et al.*, 1973). In a study of women attending a general practice in Scotland, 48% reported flushing episodes close to the time of menopause; the peak incidence occurred during the first 2 postmenopausal years (Table 1.1). Some 11% of women began flushing shortly before menopause. A similar pattern of results was obtained from a Dutch population, though the incidence of symptoms was somewhat higher (Jaszmann *et al.*, 1969a). Flushing has been claimed to be a specific symptom of the

TABLE 1.1

Vasomotor Instability (Flushing Experience) of Women in Aberdeen[a]

Menopausal status	Flushing			Number of women
	Current	Stopped	Never	
Premenopausal	11	—	87	98
Menopausal	6	1	9	16
Postmenopausal	37	41	29	107
Years since menopause				
<2	11	2	1	14
2–3	7	2	1	10
3–4	4	3	1	8
4–6	8	7	11	26
7–9	5	11	8	24
≥10	1	15	7	23
Not stated	1	1	—	2
Total number of women	54	42	125	221

[a] From Thompson *et al.* (1973).

menopause because it is observed so consistently. Certainly it is highly responsive to exogenous oestrogens. On the other hand, several of the 11 climacteric symptoms listed in Kupperman's Index (Kupperman *et al.*, 1959) have been found to respond in some studies (Hagen *et al.*, 1982a), but some benefits are probably indirect. The relationship between endogenous oestrogens and the occurrence of these symptoms is not as clear-cut as hormone replacement studies would suggest because levels of oestrone and oestradiol are not necessarily lower in symptomatic women compared with asymptomatic women (p. 127). The biological bases of the major symptoms of the climacteric and postmenopause are described in Chapter 6.

1.5. Age at Natural Menopause

Until relatively recently few surveys of the normal age at menopause had been rigorously designed and analysed. Much of the early information was anecdotal or obtained by recall in small samples. The first large-scale study was carried out in the United Kingdom by the Medical Women's Federation in 1933.

There are many pitfalls when designing surveys for this purpose, and they are reviewed admirably by Gray (1976). Most data show that the age distribution for natural menopause is broad and negatively skewed (i.e. a wider scatter of women at lower menopausal ages) (Fig. 1.3). The asymmetrical distribution results in mean values which are sometimes as much as 2 or 3 years less than the medians (Table 1.2). Most authors now choose medians to express their results since this parameter (the 50th centile) is a more meaningful indication of the central tendency of a population. The median is generally calculated by estimating the percentage of postmenopausal women at each age and transforming the percentages into probits or logits to make the distribution more symmetrical. The median is then calculated from the probit or logit mean (Finney, 1971).

No refinements of analytic technique can compensate for poor data. Surveys have often been based on selected populations (e.g. through a hospital or general

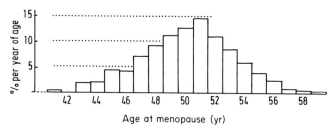

Fig. 1.3. Frequency distribution of age at menopause among American white women ($n = 393$). (From Treloar, 1981; reprinted with permission.)

TABLE 1.2

Estimated Age of the Human Menopause

Country and year of study	Race	Age at menopause (years)		Study design	References
		Mean	Median		
Australia, 1978	Caucasian		50.4	Cross-sectional	Walsh (1978)
Czechoslovakia, 1967	Caucasian		49.03	Retrospective	Magursky et al. (1975)
England, 1951–1961	Caucasian		49.82	Cross-sectional	Frommer (1964)
1965	Caucasian		50.78	Cross-sectional	McKinlay et al. (1972)
Finland, 1961	Caucasian	47.49		Retrospective	Hauser et al. (1961)
Germany (FDR), 1972	Caucasian	49.8		Retrospective	Hofmann and Soergel (1972)
India (Punjab), 1966	Asian	49.06	44.0	Cohort and cross-sectional	Wyon et al. (1966)
1975	Asian	44.68		Retrospective	Singh and Ahuja (1980)
Israel, 1963	Caucasian	49.5		Retrospective	Hauser et al. (1963)
Mexico, 1968–1978	American Indian	40.4		Retrospective	Chavez and Martinez (1982)
Netherlands, 1969	Caucasian	51.4		Cross-sectional	Jaszmann et al. (1969b)
1977	Caucasian		51.7	Retrospective	van Keep et al. (1979)
New Zealand, 1967	Caucasian		50.7	Cross-sectional	Burch and Gunz (1967)
Papua New Guinea, 1973	Melanesian		47.3 (Not malnourished)	Cross-sectional	Scragg (1973)
			43.6 (Malnourished)		
Scotland, 1970	Caucasian		50.1	Cross-sectional	Thompson et al. (1973)
South Africa, 1960	Negro	47.7	48.1	Retrospective	Abramson et al. (1960)
1960	Caucasian	48.7	49.7	Retrospective	Benjamin (1960)
1971	Negro		50.4	Cross-sectional	Frere (1971)
1971	Caucasian		49.6	Cross-sectional	Frere (1971)
Sweden, 1968–1969	Caucasian		50.4	Retrospective and cross-sectional	Bengtsson et al. (1981)
1974–1975	Caucasian		49.8		
Switzerland, 1961	Caucasian	49.8		Retrospective	Hauser et al. (1961)
United States, 1934–1974	Caucasian	49.5	49.31	Cohort	Treloar (1974)
1966	Negro		49.31	Cross-sectional	MacMahon and Worcester (1966)
1966	Caucasian		50.02	Cross-sectional	MacMahon and Worcester (1966)

practice) rather than on random samples. Furthermore, many early studies were retrospective and therefore subject to inaccurate recall and unconscious bias. There was a tendency to round up estimates to the nearest 0 or 5, which led to an artifically high incidence of menopause at ages 40, 45 and 50 years (MacMahon and Worcester, 1966; McKinlay *et al.,* 1972). Furthermore, most women recall only the year of their menopause and not the date, leading to further loss of precision. The net effect of these inaccuracies is a variable, but significant, underestimation of the age of menopause (Gray, 1976). The precision of recall in questionnaires has been studied by verifying the results with an independent source (Bean *et al.,* 1979). Here 75% of women were accurate to ±1 year, but the results might have been less reassuring if the sample had been obtained from a less well-educated and less motivated population.

Most modern surveys take account of these design problems. Two methods are commonly used: (1) *cross-sectional study design,* in which age and menopausal status are determined at the time of interview and (2) *longitudinal cohort design,* in which groups of women are studied until they reach their natural menopause. However, even these designs are not free from bias since, for example, early menopause is more likely to be represented than very late menopause if there is an upper age limit for the study. Nevertheless, a great deal of useful data has been obtained through surveys. Most studies have found median ages of menopause between 49 and 51 in Western nations (Table 1.2).

Once the normal age of menopause has been established, attempts can be made to identify biological and sociological variables. Some variables that may affect menopausal age are discussed below.

Genetic Factors. It is undoubtedly true that the size of the ovarian follicle endowment laid down in the fetus and the rate of subsequent follicle utilization and death are under genetic control. This is particularly evident in some mutant mice and in chromosomally abnormal women in whom few follicles are found (p. 56). However, there are no studies of twins or families to assess critically the contribution of genetics to the normal variation of menopausal age. Despite assertions that menopause occurs later in northern and Anglo-Saxon peoples than in other populations (Flint, 1976), there is no proof that heritable factors are responsible. In the United States and South Africa, median menopausal ages of Negroid and Caucasian subpopulations differ by less than a year (Table 1.2). In some developing countries the onset of menopause is much earlier. Menopause occurs at age 44 in Punjabis of India (Wyon *et al.,* 1966; Singh and Ahuja, 1980), at 43 or 47 in the different groups of the Bundi sub-population of Papua, New Guinea (Scragg, 1973), and at 40 in Mexican Indians (Chavez and Martinez, 1982). Such data might be accounted for by genetic isolation, but they can be explained more convincingly on other grounds, as indicated in the following sections.

Nutrition, Body Size and Composition. The lower menopausal ages of women in developing nations have often been attributed to a poor diet. In support of this hypothesis, the age of menopause was lower amongst malnourished women (43.6) than amongst those who were better nourished in Papua, New Guinea (47.3) (Scragg, 1973). Moreover, in well-nourished women there is an association between the percentage of body fat early in adulthood and the age of menopause (Sherman *et al.*, 1981). Early nutritional adequacy seems to maximize the length of menstrual life. Other studies in the United States and The Netherlands showed that women who were lean and had small statures tended to have an earlier menopause (MacMahon and Worcester, 1966; van Keep *et al.*, 1979). However, the effects of undernutrition on menopause are not as firmly established as are those on menarcheal age and length of lactational amenorrhoea (Bongaarts, 1980). Nor is it clear how severe and chronic undernutrition/malnutrition might cause early menopause. It is widely assumed that a poor diet will always be detrimental to reproduction, yet feeding mice only on alternate days has been found to delay the loss of oocytes and increase the age at which ovarian cycles cease after restoration to a normal diet (Nelson *et al.*, 1985). These effects are associated with the generally improved physiological robustness and longevity of calorie-restricted rodents, but it is not clear whether they apply to our species. Rather than looking for factors that accelerate follicular atresia in the postnatal human ovary, we should pay more attention to the developing organ. Poorly nourished women are likely to have been delivered by mothers who were similarly deprived for at least at some seasons of the year when food shortages and a high agriculture workload leads to a negative energy balance. This situation may have adversely affected fetal oogonia during their limited period of proliferation, leading to a small follicular store at the beginning of life.

Socio-Economic Factors and the Secular Trend. The historical change in socio-economic conditions and the associated improvement in nutrition and somatic growth are responsible for the advancing age of menarche in Western nations (Fig. 1.4). This downward trend, which formerly proceeded at the rate of about 0.3 years per decade, has now halted in several of these countries where the mean menarcheal age is about 13 years (Tanner, 1978). For similar reasons, it has been claimed that the age of menopause has become delayed in recent history (Backman, 1948; Frommer, 1964), although the data are questionable and subsequent studies have not confirmed a secular trend (Burch and Gunz, 1967; McKinlay *et al.*, 1972; Bengtsson, 1979; van Keep *et al.*, 1979). The ages of menarche and menopause have not been found to be correlated in most population surveys, notwithstanding the extension at both ends of menstrual life in short, fatter women (see the section on "Nutrition, Body Size and Composition" above). There is some evidence that menopause occurs earlier in women of low social class and lower income (MacMahon and Worcester, 1966; Soberon *et*

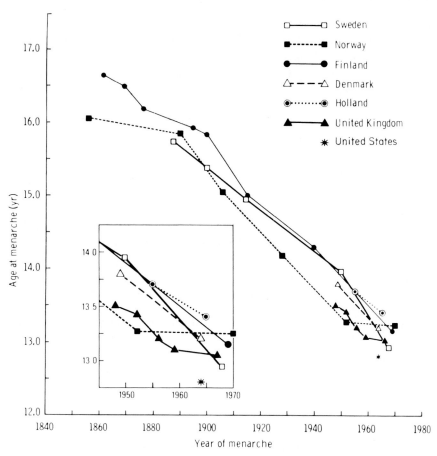

Fig. 1.4. Secular decline in age of menarche in developed countries, 1860–1970. (From Tanner, 1978; reprinted with permission.)

al., 1966), but the differences are small and have not been observed consistently (Jaszmann *et al.*, 1969b; Thompson *et al.*, 1973).

Marital Status. Single women may reach menopause slightly earlier than married women. This effect is not accounted for by associated variables such as parity (Jaszmann *et al.*, 1969b; McKinlay *et al.*, 1972; Magursky *et al.*, 1975; Brand and Lehert, 1978).

Parity. The relationship between the number of pregnancies and menopausal age is controversial, and there have been several negative findings (Medical Women's Federation, 1933; Frommer, 1964; MacMahon and Worcester, 1966;

Jaszmann *et al.*, 1969b; Thompson *et al.*, 1973; Walsh, 1978; Ernster and Petrakis, 1981). Some of the controversy can be traced to the complex relationship between this variable and socio-economic factors. In two studies, one in London and the other in Mexico City, there was evidence that high parity was associated with later menopause in the high-income group but not in the low-income group (Soberon *et al.*, 1966; McKinlay *et al.*, 1972). At one time, high parity was thought to exhaust reproductive potential and possibly to advance menopause, but this hypothesis finds no convincing support (Flint, 1976). In addition, the contrary hypothesis that oocytes are used more parsimoniously and therefore conserved during pregnancy has no biological foundation (p. 50). Any effects of parity on menopausal age are more likely to be due to socio-economic factors.

Contraceptive Practice. Since the endometrium is sensitive to ovarian steroids even in extreme old age, oral contraceptives can conceal the transition to the postmenopause. Long-term contraceptive practice during the fertile years of life would not be expected to conserve oocytes for the same reason parity does not. Epidemiological studies have, however, found a slightly later median age of menopause according to consumption of contraceptive pills (van Keep *et al.*, 1979). This surprising finding requires confirmation. There are no obvious reasons why any other contraceptive method should affect the timing of ovarian failure. In an Israeli study, menopause occurred at younger ages among women who had had many abortions (Pumpianski, 1967). This remarkable claim also requires close study.

Geography and Climate. As already stated, the menopausal age of women in tropical countries has been reported to be lower than that in boreal regions of the world. The effects of climate, if any, are likely to be indirect. Similarly, it is unlikely that living at altitudes above 2000–3000 m compared with lower altitudes in Chile and India has either a direct or specific effect on the time of menopause (Flint, 1976).

Smoking. Cigarette smoking has been associated with earlier menopause in a number of developed countries (Jick *et al.*, 1977; van Keep *et al.*, 1979; Lindquist and Bengtsson, 1979; Kaufman *et al.*, 1980). The differences in menopausal age between women who had never smoked and those who had smoked >14 cigarettes per day since age 35 years or less was almost 2 years in one multicentre study (Table 1.3). These results are important because additional years of postmenopause aggravate the risk of fractured bones and other problems later in life (see Section 6.3). Tobacco smoke and tar constituents may exert many subtle effects on the function of ovaries. They have adverse effects on blood vessel walls and reduce the oxygen-carrying capacity of haemoglobin. It has even been suggested that they might affect neuroendocrine function and steroid metabo-

TABLE 1.3

Mean Age at Menopause among 656 Naturally Postmenopausal Women Aged 60–69 According to the Number of Cigarettes Smoked (Data from the United States, Canada and Israel)[a]

Number of cigarettes[b]	Number of women	Mean age at menopause (years)	Mean difference from never-smokers (years)	SE of difference
Never-smoker	434	49.4	—	—
Ex-smoker	10	49.2	0.2	1.5
1–14/day	66	48.0	1.4	0.6
15–24/day	99	47.6	1.8	0.5
≥25/day	47	47.6	1.8	0.7

[a] From Kaufman *et al.* (1980).

[b] Smoking status at the time of the interview. All smokers began smoking before age 35; all ex-smokers stopped smoking before age 35.

lism, further compromising the function of the ageing ovary. One product of smoking materials which is also present in urban air pollution, benzo(a)pyrene, might actually reduce the size of the follicular reserve because small amounts can kill mouse oocytes (Mattison and Thorgeirsson, 1978). Other smoking materials may also affect menopause, although surveys have not been conducted because these materials are used clandestinely in many places. Of particular interest is marihuana because of its widespread use and the reported effects of the chief psychoactive constituent, tetrahydrocannabinol, on reproductive functions, including pulsatile release of pituitary luteinizing hormone (LH) (Tyrey, 1980).

Disease and Drugs. A number of diseases are associated with altered (usually earlier) menopause (Flint, 1976), but it is difficult to distinguish the effects of advanced or chronic illness from iatrogenic effects. This subject is discussed further in a later section (Section 3.7).

In conclusion, the menopause is a universal characteristic of women, occurring at a median age of about 49–51 years in well-nourished societies. The estimated ages are remarkably consistent in view of the diversity of diets, life styles and environments of the peoples that have been studied. The explanation of menopause is therefore firmly in the province of the biologist.

1.6. Menopause in Animals

There is a bewildering array of physiological strategies for reproduction in mammals, and even closely related species have sometimes evolved quite differently in this respect. Only in monkeys of the Old World and in the great apes do we find menstrual cycles fairly similar in length and endocrinology to those of women. Strictly speaking, only these species can serve as potential models for studying human menstrual cycles and menopause.

Unequivocal evidence of spontaneous menopause has been obtained only in captive colonies of rhesus monkeys (*Macaca mulatta*). The menopause occurs between 20 and 30 years of age (i.e. close to the maximum longevity under these conditions) and is followed by hormonal changes that are consistent with primary ovarian failure (van Wagenen, 1972; Hodgen *et al.*, 1977; Diershke *et al.*, 1983). Pigtail macaques (*M. nemestrina*) may reach menopause at similar ages (Graham *et al.*, 1979). The natural fertility pattern of great apes might be expected to resemble the human pattern even more closely. However, despite the greater longevity (c. 50 years), chimpanzees continue to show cycles until death, although they fail to conceive at advanced ages (Graham, 1979). Tentative signs of menopause have recently been recorded in two extremely old chimpanzees (*Pan troglodytes*) and in one pigmy chimpanzee (*P. paniscus*) at the Yerkes Primate Center (Gould *et al.*, 1981). Despite limited data, it seems safe to state that a postmenopausal phase of life is relatively short and confined to a few animals of exceptional longevity under present husbandry conditions. The rarity of all apes and, to a lesser extent, monkeys, combined with the costs and patience required for keeping them until advanced age, are major limitations for menopause research.

Rodents are a poor compromise when animal models are needed for analysing certain aspects of ageing in the human reproductive system. Since rodents do not have menstrual cycles, they cannot *ipso facto* become menopausal, although many exhibit a prolonged postreproductive phase beginning at mid-life. No specific term has yet been coined for this phase; the neologism "oestropause" is superficially attractive but fails to convey the variety of endocrine and behaviour patterns of postcyclic life, which rarely find parallels in human biology. Despite some contrasting patterns of ageing in rodents and primates, which will be described further, the former will continue to be important models for tackling the most fundamental biological questions.

2

Oestrogen—Queen of the Realm of Reproduction

2.1. Discovery and Characterization

Present knowledge of the chemistry and biology of oestrogens is based upon discoveries made at the turn of this century, although Chinese chemists had obtained urinary preparations of oestrogens much earlier. In 1896, Knauer established the endocrine activity of ovaries by showing that the effects of castration were reversed by ovarian grafts. Marshall and Jolly (1906) proposed that follicular or interstitial ovarian cells are responsible for oestrous phenomena in animals, but they had no means of purifying the hormones. The first clues to the chemical identity and source of oestrogens were obtained by Allen and Doisy (1923), who found that extracts of porcine follicular fluid had trophic effects on the genital tracts of ovariectomized rats. During the following decade, the most important discoveries were made by chemists who eventually characterized and synthesized the major ovarian steroids (see Doisy, 1972, and Butenandt and Westphal, 1974, for historical accounts).

Early attempts to isolate oestrogens were hampered by the limited amounts of hormones in porcine ovaries, but progress quickened when much larger quantities were found in the urine of pregnant women. In 1929, Doisy and Butenandt, working independently in the United States and Germany, respectively, obtained pure crystalline steroids and concluded that oestrone (called "theelin" in those times) was a hydroxyketone with the formula $C_{18}H_{22}O_2$. The following year in London, Marrian identified another oestrogen called "theelol", which later became known as "oestriol". Identification of a third oestrogen (oestradiol-17β or "dihydrotheelin") was delayed until 1936 because of low tissue concentrations. Doisy's group eventually recovered 6 mg of the pure substance from a ton of porcine ovaries (MacCorquodale et al., 1936). Nearly a quarter of a century elapsed before this was shown to be the principal oestrogen of human ovaries (Zander et al., 1959). Meanwhile, vast amounts of animal tissue were being extracted to obtain crystalline progesterone and male sex hormones, which were identified in the early 1930s.

The natural oestrogens are a small family of molecules within the nation of steroids. The structures of the three classical oestrogens named above are shown in Fig. 2.1. They have in common the biological property of stimulating uterine growth and vaginal cornification in rodents (and other species). This characteristic defines all oestrogens, natural and synthetic. Their biological potency differs. Oestrone is only 15–25% as potent as oestradiol in bioassays, although comparisons are difficult because of interconversion in tissue. Single injections of oestriol are not uterotrophic because the nuclear receptor–oestriol complex is retained for only a short period, but continuous administration can result in normal oestrogenic responses (Anderson et al., 1975).

Urine of pregnant mares is another rich source of sex steroids. Besides the classical oestrogens, it contains specific oestrogens, equilin and equilenin, in which the B ring of the steroid nucleus is unsaturated (Fig. 2.1). Conjugated equine oestrogens are of therapeutic importance for climacteric and postmenopausal symptoms because they are readily absorbed from the gut and join the systemic circulation. A currently popular formulation used in the United States and, to less extent, in the United Kingdom consists of oestrone sulphate (48%), equilin sulphate (26%) and 17α-dihydroequilin sulphate (15%) with other conjugated oestrogens in small amounts ("Premarin") (Hammond and Maxson, 1982).

Since natural unconjugated oestrogens are relatively inactive after ingestion, new compounds have been sought. The first orally active oestrogen that became widely available is not a steroid but a stilbene derivative, diethylstilboestrol (Dodds et al., 1938). During the same period, the Schering Corporation found that oestradiol became orally active when an ethinyl group was attached to the

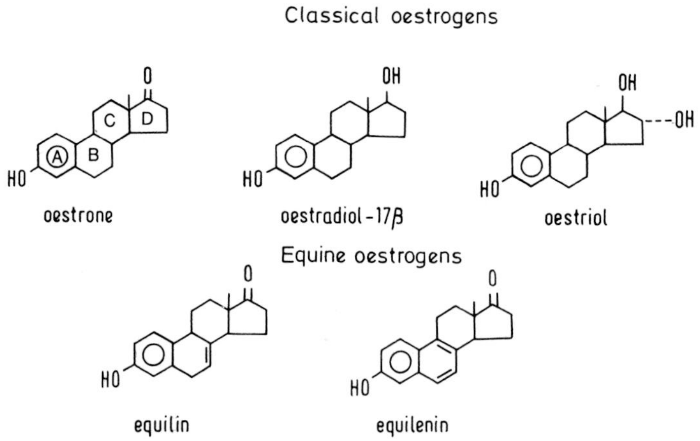

Fig. 2.1. Structure of natural oestrogens, showing standard nomenclature of carbon rings in steroid nucleus (A, B, C, D).

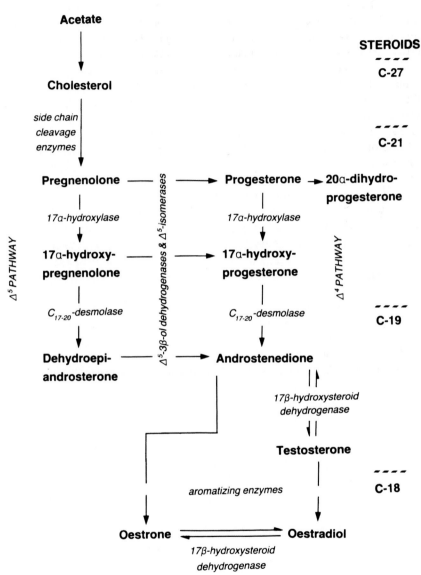

Fig. 2.2. Major pathways for biosynthesis of oestrogens in the ovary.

C-17 position on the molecule. These were the first of many discoveries of practical importance.

When the structures of steroid hormones were elucidated, it was apparent that these substances might be derived from cholesterol. This hypothesis was confirmed when deuterium was shown to be transferred from cholesterol to pregnanediol in pregnant women (Bloch, 1945). Subsequently, the availability of steroids labelled with ^{14}C and ^{3}H at high specific activity led to rapid progress in unravelling the biosynthetic pathway for oestrogen formation (Fig. 2.2). Side chain cleavage of cholesterol, involving at least three enzymes, leads to a C-21 steroid, pregnenolone, which is the precursor of the three main classes of ovarian steroids, namely, progestogens, androgens and oestrogens. That androgens are normal intermediaries in the biosynthesis of oestrogens was first indicated by the formation of oestrogen after administration of testosterone propionate to men (Steinach and Kun, 1937). Biochemical studies demonstrated that, although the ovary and placenta are the major sites of oestrogen production in women, a number of tissues have the ability to produce oestrogens. Aromatization of C-19 androgens to form phenolic C-18 oestrogens occurs in a specific cellular fraction containing the microsomes and is catalysed by a mixed-function oxidase in the presence of nicotinamide adenosine dinucleotide phosphate (NADPH) and molecular oxygen (Ryan, 1959).

The title of this chapter is adapted from words of F. L. Hisaw and signifies the central role of the oestrogens in the realm of sexual physiology and behaviour. Oestrogens are pre-eminently responsible for the sex-specific form and physiology of female mammals. They are essential for fertility, and widespread metabolic consequences follow their withdrawal. Few, if any, other groups of hormones match the oestrogens for biological potency on a molar basis or in the range of cell types affected. For these reasons, and because they are deficient in the postmenopause, they have been singled out for special consideration.

2.2. Production of Ovarian Oestrogen

The ovary is the main site of oestrogen production during menstrual and oestrous cycles. Lower blood hormone levels after castration and menopause are clear evidence of this. It is much less certain which ovarian cells are responsible for synthesizing oestrogens. At one time the theca interna of follicles was held responsible, but subsequent research tended to uphold the suggestion that "all ovarian tissues may secrete oestrogen . . . but that the follicular epithelium is the primary source" (Allen, 1941).

Leaving aside for a moment the vexed question of the site of production, let us examine some general requirements for biosynthesis of oestradiol-17β (henceforward called "oestradiol"), the principal oestrogen of ovarian cycles in women and most animals. Maturation of Graafian follicles and maximal production of oestradiol occur at the same phase of the cycle and depend on gonadotrophic hormones from the pituitary gland. Optimal trophic responses in ovaries of hypophysectomized rats require follicle-stimulating hormone (FSH) and luteinizing hormone (LH) in combination (Lostroh and Johnson, 1966; Armstrong and Papkoff, 1976). The levels of gonadotrophins are controlled, in turn, by inhibitory and stimulatory feedback by steroids and, perhaps, by non-steroidal products of the ovary to bring about the normal sequences of growth, ovulation and luteinization (Fig. 2.3).

Growing follicles possess specific receptors of high affinity for FSH and LH in their cell membranes. The receptors are distributed unevenly. FSH receptors are found exclusively in granulosa cells, whereas LH receptors are present in theca cells, though appearing in granulosa cells during final stages of preovulatory maturation (Richards, 1979). Binding of gonadotrophins to their receptors initi-

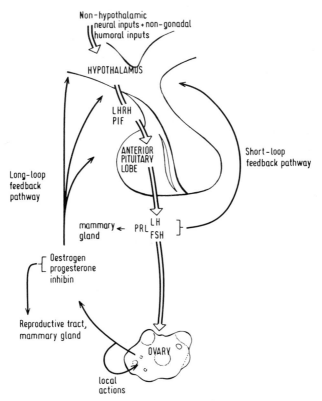

Fig. 2.3. Neuroendocrine regulation of ovarian function: summary of major pathways and feedback. LHRH, luteinizing hormone releasing hormone; PIF, prolactin inhibiting factor; PRL, prolactin; FSH, follicle-stimulating hormone.

ates a chain of biochemical events. There is a conformational change in the hormone–receptor complex which allows binding to a regulatory protein and, hence, activation of adenylate cyclase. This enzyme catalyses conversion of adenosine triphosphate (ATP) to cyclic adenosine $3'$, $5'$-monophosphate (cyclic AMP), which can phosphorylate protein kinases and bring about observable biological effects: growth, differentiation and secretion. Thus, interactions between gonadotrophins and their ovarian target cells lead indirectly to the many physiological changes of ovarian cycles.

There is substantial evidence that the rising levels of oestradiol produced by the dominant follicle(s) require cooperation of theca and granulosa cells. Falck (1959) isolated these cells from rat follicles by microdissection and transplanted them to the anterior chamber of the eye, together with vaginal epithelium to act as an oestrogen indicator. They produced oestrogen only when they were present together.

Short (1962) proposed a different mechanism of oestradiol production based on measurements of hormone levels in equine follicular fluid and luteal tissue. He suggested that the theca interna produces oestrogens and androgens, whereas luteinized granulosa cells produce progesterone. The ability of corpora lutea of some species (e.g. humans) to secrete oestradiol could then be explained by the presence of theca lutein cells. Short coined the term "two-cell type" theory, but this term is now also used to describe different mechanisms of oestrogen biosynthesis in other species.

Confirmation of Falck's results has now been obtained from studies of rodents by combining the practical advantages of tissue culture with the precision of hormone radioimmunoassay. Theca cells released mainly androgens, and their secretory activity was increased by human chorionic gonadotrophin (hCG)/LH (but not FSH). Isolated granulosa cells tended to luteinize spontaneously and produced large quantities of progesterone but very little androgen or oestrogen. When the two cell types were combined in short-term experiments, larger amounts of oestradiol were formed (Makris and Ryan, 1975; Fortune and Armstrong, 1977). Other studies show granulosa cells possess aromatase (oestrogen synthetase), which is stimulated in a dose-dependent manner by FSH in the presence of testosterone (Dorrington et al., 1975; Erickson and Hsueh, 1978). Since this stimulation is blocked by actinomycin D and by cycloheximide, it is presumed that enzyme induction/activation involves de novo synthesis of RNA and protein (Wang et al., 1982). These results have been interpreted to mean that androgens (androstenedione and testosterone) synthesized in the theca interna under the control of LH diffuse into the follicle, where they are converted to oestradiol by granulosa cells primed by FSH.

This model of oestradiol production in rodent follicles has been called the "two-cell, two-gonadotrophin theory" (Armstrong et al., 1979) (Fig. 2.4). It is presumably based on a differential distribution of enzymes. Non-luteinized granulosa cells contain aromatase but are deficient in 17α-hydroxylase and C_{17-20^-}

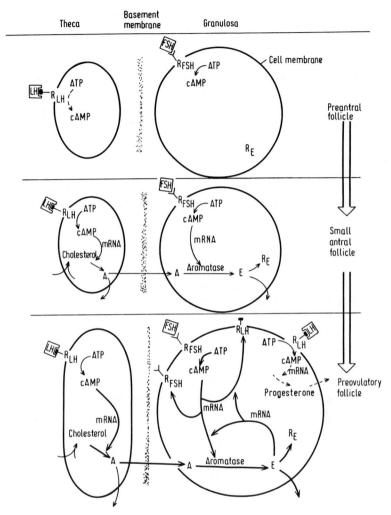

Fig. 2.4. Schematic diagram of ovarian follicular biosynthesis of oestrogen by co-operation of theca interna and granulosa cells. Aromatizable androgens (A) are synthesized in the theca layer in the presence of LH stimulation. They diffuse to the granulosa layer, where they are substrates for aromatization to oestrogen (E) in the presence of FSH. The gonadotrophins exert their actions by a chain of events: binding to receptors (R) in cell membranes, which leads to increasing intracellular levels of cyclic AMP (cAMP) and enzyme induction/activation. FSH and oestrogen have synergistic effects of inducing LH receptors in preovulatory follicles which increasingly produce progesterone. FSH receptors increase during follicle growth *pari passu* with granulosa cell number, although they may decrease later.

desmolase, which are obligatory for converting C-21 steroids to androgens in the Δ4 pathway. This deficiency is compensated for by the acquisition of enzymes by theca cells during Graafian follicle development (Bogovich and Richards, 1982).

This model is consistent with data obtained for some other species. Moor (1977) showed that theca cells were the source of androgens in cultured sheep follicles and that co-culture with granulosa cells was required for the formation of significant amounts of oestradiol. Direct evidence of the two-cell theory was obtained in the same species by Baird (1977a). He found oestrogen secretion from the ovary carrying the dominant (ovulable) follicle was inhibited >50% after infusing antiserum to testosterone into the ovarian artery. Since antibodies do not normally enter cells, the results imply that androgens leave cells before they are aromatized.

There are data in other species which are inconsistent with this model. As implied above, there are strong indications that theca cells are responsible for oestradiol formation in equine follicles (YoungLai and Short, 1970). In addition, when radioactively labelled acetate was presented to human granulosa and theca cells in vitro, all steroid intermediaries between cholesterol and oestrogens were recovered (Ryan et al., 1968). Oestrogens were produced via the Δ4 pathway in the granulosa cells, whereas Δ5 was the preferred pathway of theca cells (Ryan and Petro, 1966) (Fig. 2.2). Similar differentiation of the two cell types is seen in rabbit follicles (Patwardhan and Lanthier, 1977). Although these experiments show the presence of enzymes, it does not follow that these pathways are necessarily operating in vivo. To help answer this question, granulosa cells and follicular fluid were aspirated from dominant follicles in rhesus monkeys (Channing and Coudert, 1976). The levels of oestrogens in blood draining from the ovaries were hardly affected by this treatment, suggesting that the theca was responsible for secretion. A problem with this type of experiment is that peripheral granulosa cells probably make the major contribution to oestrogen production (Zoller and Weisz, 1978) and are the most difficult to remove. Nevertheless, it seems probable that there are genuine species differences in the biosynthetic role of various ovarian cell types.

Although far from decisive, there is some evidence of two-cell co-operation for the production of oestrogen by human ovaries. Isolated human theca cells have limited aromatase activity: they produce <1% of the amount of oestrogen produced by granulosa cells from the same follicles (Moon et al., 1978; McNatty et al., 1979a; Hillier et al., 1981). When combined in vitro, the two cell types produce more oestrogen than the sum of their independent production (Batta et al., 1980). Theca cells resemble their stroma cell precursors both in this respect and in their ability to secrete quantities of androstenedione and testosterone. Thecal androgen secretion rises during the follicular phase and is greater than that of an equivalent mass of stroma. However, the large bulk of stroma implies a substantial contribution to total ovarian production (McNatty et al., 1979a).

The ability of human ovarian follicles to produce oestrogen rises during the follicular phase because of the increased size and heightened aromatase activity in individual granulosa cells. Indeed, follicles that are presumed to be healthy and progressing towards ovulation are identified by large amounts of oestradiol in follicular fluid, rising to 2.5 µg/ml. Androgen levels in preovulatory follicles become less predominant, but the rate of aromatization is not limited by lack of substrate (McNatty and Baird, 1978).

The largest healthy follicle measures 5–8 mm in diameter at the beginning of the menstrual cycle (Gougeon and Lefèvre, 1983) and contains FSH and oestradiol in its fluid (McNatty and Baird, 1978). The relatively high levels of plasma FSH at this stage promote aromatase activity (Erickson et al., 1979). Oestradiol production is self-reinforcing. It causes proliferation of granulosa cells (Rao et al., 1978); consequently, healthy follicles have more granulosa cells than non-ovulatory follicles of similar diameter (McNatty et al., 1979b), and the numbers of FSH receptors rise correspondingly. Oestradiol also promotes aromatase activity within cells (Fig. 2.4). These actions help protect the dominant follicle(s) from understimulation during the second half of the follicular phase, when levels of plasma FSH fall (Fig. 3.5), by increasing both the efficiency of trapping FSH and the sensitivity of granulosa cells. By this time, the follicle exceeds 12 mm in diameter, and increasing production of oestrogen may depend on pronounced LH pulses to stimulate greater production of androgen (Bäckström et al., 1982). Furthermore, as rat follicles approach ovulation, they become much more sensitive to the stimulatory effects of LH on the production of cyclic AMP and oestradiol (Uilenbroek and Richards, 1979). Such responsiveness is likely to follow the acquisition of LH receptors on granulosa cells, which depends on the joint action of FSH and oestradiol (Richards, 1979). Subsequently, these cells become increasingly active in producing progesterone, anticipating their morphological transformation to luteal cells.

Non-ovulatory follicles do not not develop FSH-sensitive aromatase activity and do not therefore switch from androgen to oestrogen production (McNatty et al., 1979a; Mori et al., 1982). Androgen production continues during early stages of atresia (McNatty et al., 1979a). Androgens serve a complex role in follicular maturation; besides being obligatory precursors of oestrogens, they are also evidently involved in priming granulosa cells for induction/activation of aromatase by FSH (Hillier and de Zwart, 1981). Other experiments show that androgens can inhibit aromatase, and they have even been held responsible for atresia (Louvet et al., 1975). More research is required to clarify their role.

Increasing output of ovarian steroids during the first half of the cycle is a sign of follicular growth, whereas the changing profile of hormones represented (androgens to oestrogens to progestogens) is indicative of cellular differentiation and maturation in the dominant follicle. Since some circulating oestrogen is derived from extra-ovarian sources, it is useful to measure its blood production rate (BPR), the total production from all sources, glandular and extra-glandular

TABLE 2.1

Ovarian Steroids during the Menstrual Cycle and following Menopause: Representative Blood Production Rates, Plasma Concentrations and Metabolic Clearance Rates

Steroid	Blood production rate (mg/24 hr)				Peripheral plasma concentration (pg/ml)				Metabolic clearance rate (litres of plasma/24 hr)		References
	EF[a]	MC[b]	ML[c]	PMP[d]	EF[a]	MC[b]	ML[c]	PMP[d]	M[e]	PMP[d]	
Oestradiol	0.074	0.429	0.258	0.006	55	318	191	7	1350	910	Baird and Fraser (1974) Baird and Guevara (1969) Korenman et al. (1969) Longcope (1971) Longcope et al. (1968) Siiteri and MacDonald (1973)
Oestrone	0.133	0.265	0.236	0.040	60	120	107	25	2210	1610	
Androstenedione	2.91	4.60	3.75	1.70	1450	2290	1870	930	2010	1830	Abraham (1974) Baird et al. (1974) Grodin et al. (1973)
Testosterone	0.152	0.345	0.207	0.150	220	500	300	300	690	500	Judd and Yen (1973) Siiteri and MacDonald (1973) Tait and Horton (1966) Vermeulen (1976)
Progesterone	0.682	4.44	31.13	—	310	2000	14150	190	2200	—	Johansson (1969) Vermeulen (1976)

[a] EF, early follicular phase.
[b] MC, mid-cycle.
[c] ML, mid-luteal phase.
[d] PMP, postmenopause.
[e] M, menstrual cycle.

(mg/24 hr). The BPR can be obtained indirectly by measuring the metabolic clearance rate (MCR) of the hormone. The MCR is the volume of plasma completely and irreversibly cleared of hormone in unit time (litres per 24 hr). This is estimated by infusing radioactively labelled hormone into a peripheral vein until blood concentrations are stable. At this point, the rate of infusion balances the rate of removal or metabolism, and the MCR can be calculated. The BPR is then obtained as the product of the MCR and the plasma hormone concentration.

The BPR of oestradiol rises from 0.03 mg/24 hr at menstruation to about 0.40 mg/24 hr shortly before ovulation (Table 2.1). Comparisons between peripheral and ovarian vein blood indicate about 95% of peak levels are formed by the "active" ovary containing the dominant follicle in monovular cycles (Baird,1977b). Very little oestradiol is secreted by the human adrenal gland or formed extra-glandularly. Consequently, it has been concluded that "in reproductively active women estradiol is secreted almost exclusively from the preovulatory follicle or the corpus luteum, and the blood production rate equals the secretion rate" (Baird, 1977b). Plasma levels of oestrone are similar to those of oestradiol, but cyclical variations are less marked because of a greater extra-ovarian contribution (Baird and Guevara, 1969). The ovary may also secrete oestrone sulphate, but secretion of oestriol has not been established (Baird, 1978).

Larger quantities of androgens than oestrogens are produced at all stages of the ovarian cycle (Table 2.1). Besides circulating as prohormones, they probably have important (but presently undefined) physiological actions and, in excess, can produce masculinization. Androstenedione is by far the most abundant ovarian androgen in ovarian vein blood, where its level exceeds that of peripheral blood levels by 20:1. Testosterone and dehydroepiandrosterone (DHEA) are also products of the ovary, judging by their fluctuating levels during the menstrual cycle and their small excess in ovarian vein blood (2:1). Plasma DHEA and androstenedione have marked diurnal rhythms, which indicates that large quantities are secreted by adrenal glands.

Progestogens are secreted in abundance by the ovary during the luteal phase. Over 90% of the BPR of progesterone (30 mg/24 hr) can be accounted for by the corpus luteum. Other C-21 steroids are secreted by follicles and corpora lutea (notably 17α-hydroxyprogesterone), but these show much less cyclical variation.

2.3. Production of Oestrogen after Menopause

In the preceding section, oestradiol was shown to be produced mainly by ovarian follicles, but few follicles remain at menopausal age (see Chapter 3). The end of menstrual life therefore marks the beginning of a new phase in which circulating oestrogen is maintained on a lower plane. During the first 6 months after menopause, significant quantities of oestrogen may be secreted intermittently (Sherman et al., 1979; Metcalf et al., 1982). Presumably, they are derived mainly from residual follicles that grow sporadically but fail to reach maturity. Subsequently, plasma oestradiol falls to low, relatively stable values of less than 20 pg/ml for the remainder of life.

The changes in rates of production of oestradiol and oestrone after menopause are not the same. The mean BPR of oestradiol in postmenopausal women is only 0.006 mg/24 hr, which is about 20% of the nadir and only 1% of mid-cycle levels of the menstrual cycle (Table 2.1). The BPR and plasma levels of oestrone fall by only about 50% to 0.04 mg/24 hr and 25 pg/ml. Oestrone is, therefore, quantitatively the most abundant oestrogen of the postmenopause, though even greater amounts of the sulphate ester are present (Roberts et al., 1980). The oestradiol:oestrone ratio in peripheral blood falls to a value that is closer to that of castrated women (0.42 ± 0.07) and men (0.35 ± 0.04) than that of menstruating women (>1.0) (Baird, 1977b).

The ovarian contribution to circulating oestrogen after menopause has been difficult to measure because of technical limitations of assaying small amounts. Even in the absence of follicles, a small contribution is expected because other ovarian tissues evidently produce small quantities in vitro (McNatty et al., 1979a). Barlow et al. (1969), using isotope dilution methods, were unable to detect any significant ovarian production. On the other hand, the concentrations of oestradiol and oestrone in ovarian vein blood were double those in peripheral blood, which suggests a residual capability for secretion (Judd et al., 1974a; Greenblatt et al., 1976). However, in another study the ovarian contribution to the circulating pool of hormones was insignificant in the majority of women (Longcope et al., 1980) and so other sources of postmenopausal oestrogen have been sought.

At first, the adrenal glands were suspected to be important sources because of long-standing evidence of sex steroid excretion in castrates (Parkes, 1937). This hypothesis seemed to be strengthened by discoveries that adrenocorticotrophic hormone (ACTH) increased urinary oestrogens, whereas adrenalectomy had the opposite effect (Dao, 1953). But measurements of adrenal vein blood indicate that, although large amounts of androgen are secreted, only small quantities of oestrone are formed and production of oestradiol is negligible (Baird et al., 1969; Greenblatt et al., 1976). Thus we are led to the conclusion that oestrogens are formed extra-glandularly.

The first clear evidence of extra-glandular production of oestrogens was obtained from two ovariectomized, adrenalectomized women in whom urinary oestrogen levels rose after injections of testosterone propionate (West et al., 1956). Later, double isotope methods provided opportunities for using elegant quantitative methods. It became possible to measure the proportion of the total amount of androgen substrate that can be converted to oestrogen, this parameter being called the conversion ratio (CR) (Siiteri and MacDonald, 1973). There is now little doubt that the bulk of oestrone in normal postmenopausal women is formed by extra-glandular conversion of androstenedione of adrenal origin (Fig. 2.5). This situation is reminiscent of the formation of oestrogens during pregnancy, in which DHEA sulphate from the fetal adrenal gland is aromatized by the placenta. However, this substrate and its unconjugated form are not converted to precursors of oestrogens in non-pregnant women (CR <0.001) (Horton and Tait, 1967) but give rise to most of the urinary 17-ketosteroids.

The CR of androstenedione to oestrone is low, but this is compensated for by an abundance of precursor. After the menopause, the BPR of androstenedione is about 1.7 mg/24 hr, which is 50% of that during the early follicular phase of premenopausal women (Table 2.1). But extra-glandular formation of oestrogens

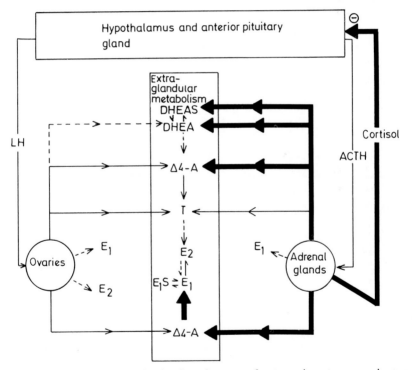

Fig. 2.5. Schematic diagram showing the major source of oestrogen in postmenopausal women. Arrows indicate direction and line thickness indicates relative activity of the pathway. Feedback by cortisol on ACTH production is indicated by $\ominus$; feedback by physiological levels of oestrogen on gonadotrophin release has not established and could be insignificant. E_1, oestrone; E_{1s}, oestrone sulphate; E_2, oestradiol; $\Delta 4\text{-}A$, androstenedione; DHEAS, dehydroepiandrosterone sulphate; T, testosterone; LH, luteinizing hormone; ACTH, corticotrophin.

does not fall correspondingly because of a rising CR. The CR is 0.013 before the menopause and 0.027 afterwards, although individual values are highly variable and probably change continuously rather than abruptly at menopause (MacDonald et al., 1967; Siiteri and MacDonald, 1973; Grodin et al., 1973). On the basis of these figures, the production rate of oestrone from androstenedione in postmenopausal women is therefore $1.7 \times 0.027 = 0.046$ mg/24 hr. Within the bounds of biological and experimental variation, this figure is not significantly different from the total BPR of oestrone obtained by other methods (0.04 mg/24 hr).

Oestrone can also be formed by peripheral conversion of androstenedione via oestradiol and testosterone (Fig. 2.5). This pathway is much less active than the alternative one because levels of testosterone are lower than those of androstenedione and because the CR for androgen to oestradiol is very low (0.001) (Longcope et al., 1969; Judd et al., 1982). Therefore, it has been concluded that most circulating oestradiol is formed by conversion of oestrone, for which the CR is more favourable (0.065) (Judd et al., 1982).

The adrenal gland is responsible for most of the circulating androstenedione and, hence, oestrone after the menopause. There are several reasons for this view. Androstenedione is not produced to any extent from extra-glandular conversion of DHEA or testosterone and must therefore be of glandular origin (Horton and Tait, 1966, 1967). Plasma levels of this androgen and those of oestrone (but not oestradiol) show a circadian rhythm that characterizes adrenal secretion; peak levels are seen at 0800 hr and a nadir occurs between 2000 hr and midnight (Vermeulen, 1976; Crilly et al., 1979). Suppression of corticotrophin (ACTH) release by corticosteroids causes plasma androstenedione levels to fall by about 50%, and there is an associated decline of oestrone (Vermeulen, 1976; Marshall et al., 1978). Similarly, plasma androgen and oestrogen levels are more than 50% lower after adrenalectomy, although testosterone is somewhat less affected if the ovaries remain (Vermeulen, 1980).

The most remarkable feature of postmenopausal oestrogen production, apart from its paucity, is its overwhelming dependence on adrenal function. The ovary has become almost redundant, and circulating oestrogen is no longer controlled by the gonadotrophins. The pituitary–gonadal feedback loop is virtually inactive. Although unproven, it is likely that exogenous oestrogen has little effect on endogenous production, in contrast to the situation in premenopausal women. Drugs or diseases that affect adrenocortical function are of considerable importance because they influence production of oestrogen substrate.

There is widespread evidence that plasma levels of five androgens fall during ageing (Zumoff et al., 1980; Meldrum et al., 1981a; Vermeulen et al., 1982) (Fig. 2.6). This cannot be explained by altered metabolic clearance rates (cf. Section 2.4) but may be due to diminished sensitivity to ACTH with less C_{17-20}-desmolase activity in the adrenal cortex. Although contrary data exist, some

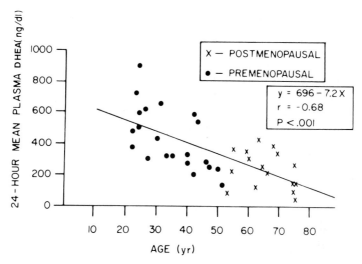

Fig. 2.6. Twenty-four-hour mean plasma dehydroepiandrosterone concentrations in normal age-ing women. (From Zumoff *et al.*, 1980; reprinted with permission.)

studies show a comparable fall of the Δ4 steroid androstenedione (Crilly *et al.*, 1979; Roger *et al.*, 1980). In some studies the changes were progressive from early adulthood, whereas in others they began shortly after menopause. Some authors have chosen the appellation ''adrenopause'' to describe these changes, which contrast with the rising androgen levels of prepuberty (''adrenarche''). Declining androgen levels are not associated with changes in cortisol production nor are they secondary to ovarian failure, since they occur in men as well as in ovariectomized women (Crilly *et al.*, 1979). The reported effects of exogenous oestrogen on adrenal androgen production are therefore probably pharmacological actions (Abraham and Maroulis, 1975). Despite these changes in androgen levels, oestrogens do not normally become more scarce during the postmenopause, and they are affected by changes in body composition rather than age *per se* (Meldrum *et al.*, 1981a).

Bilateral ovariectomy of postmenopausal women leads to lower peripheral blood levels of androgens, whereas oestrogen and progestogen levels are un-altered (Judd *et al.*, 1974b; Vermeulen, 1976; Badawy *et al.*, 1979). Androgens are the only group of steroids which rise after a large dose of hCG (Greenblatt *et al.*, 1976). The major products of the postmenopausal ovary are androgens: androstenedione, testosterone, 5α-dihydrotestosterone and, in smaller quantities, DHEA and androstenediol. The principal steroid is testosterone, judging by the 15-fold excess in blood of ovarian veins compared with that of the periphery (Judd *et al.*, 1974a). This would seem to imply that the ovary makes a significant contribution to peripheral blood levels and that testosterone is not fully accounted for by peripheral conversion of androstenedione, despite a favourable CR (~ 0.1) (Calanog *et al.*, 1977; Judd *et al.*, 1982). The excess of androstenedione in ovarian venous blood is only fourfold; therefore, indirect production of oestrogen by the ovary is small. This conclusion is supported by observations that castration does not affect oestrogen levels after menopause.

Two types of cell are probably responsible for producing most of the androgens from postmenopausal ovaries. Stroma cells contain enzymes for converting Δ5-hydroxysteroids to Δ4-ketosteroids (Fienberg, 1969) and produce androgens when isolated *in vitro* (Mattingly and Huang, 1969; McNatty *et al.*, 1979a). This activity on a unit mass basis is small but nonetheless significant because these cells are abundant and stimulated by postmenopausal gonadotrophins. Stroma cell hyperplasia and thecosis are common features of these ovaries, but they do not necessarily lead to increased androgen production (Mattingly and Huang, 1969). Hilus cells are the other important source of androgens and are found in small clusters close to the ovarian hilum (Fig. 2.7). They present the typical appearance of steroid-secreting cells, although containing cytoplasmic crystalloids of Reinke, which are found elsewhere only in human Leydig cells. Hilus cell hyperplasia and tumours lead to clinical virilization (Sternberg, 1949). Clinical evidence suggests they normally secrete testosterone and are sensitive to hCG/LH, but experimental evidence is hard to obtain because hilus cells cannot be isolated completely from stroma cells *in vitro*. Some results even suggest they produce oestrogens, but they seem anomalous and require confirmation (Dennefors *et al.*, 1982).

Differences in body size and composition of non-glandular tissues are probably responsible for much of the variation in postmenopausal oestrogen production. Knowledge of this subject is limited and animal models, which could provide impetus to basic research, have not yet been identified because most animal ovaries produce oestrogen until advanced age. The rate of production of androgens and of their conversion to oestrogens rises with excess body weight, leading to higher peripheral blood levels with an elevated oestrogen : androgen ratio (Grodin *et al.*, 1973; Edman *et al.*, 1978; Vermeulen and Verdonck, 1978; Meldrum *et al.*, 1981a), though there are contrary data (O'Dea *et al.*, 1979). Positive findings are partly explained by aromatase activity in white adipose tissue and skeletal muscle (Nimrod and Ryan, 1975; Longcope *et al.*, 1978), and wasting of these tissues in old age could account for exceptional reports that oestrogen levels decrease with increasing age postmenopause (Badawy *et al.*, 1979). Other tissues are capable of producing oestrogen in small amounts, including liver (Smuk and Schwers, 1977), bone marrow (Frisch *et al.*, 1980) and brain (Naftolin *et al.*, 1975), but the balance of production *in vivo* has not yet been measured. Excess oestrogen production in the postmenopause is associated with obesity, as well as with hepatic disease and hyperthyroidism, and may become clinically manifested with vaginal bleeding (Siiteri and MacDonald,

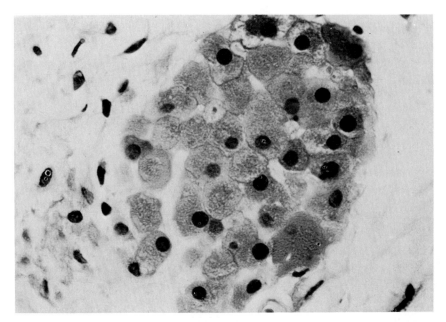

Fig. 2.7.   Nest of hilus cells in a postmenopausal human ovary. Haematoxylin and eosin (X500).

1973; Southren *et al.*, 1974). It might also lead insidiously to carcinoma of the endometrium and, perhaps, even of the breast, as obesity is known to be a risk factor for both of these diseases. There is, however, no simple connection between obesity and elevated plasma oestrogen, although associations are sometimes reported (e.g. Vermeulen, 1980), nor is there any close correlation between hormone levels and the presence of disease or the absence of climacteric symptoms. Siiteri (1981) has drawn attention to the likelihood that the free steroid fraction (which is increased in obese women) is of greater significance than total levels of oestrogen. Clearly, the factors determining oestrogenic activity in postmenopausal women are highly complex and probably change during ageing.

2.4. Metabolism and Clearance

The metabolism and clearance of the three classical oestrogens have been shown to be inter-related by *in vivo* experiments using radioactively labelled test substances. The fate of injected oestradiol is determined mainly in the liver, where it is converted to oestrone and oestriol. These products are excreted in urine after further metabolism or after conjugation with D-glucuronic acid or sulphuric acid or both. Steroid esters are more polar than free steroids and are therefore readily excreted, but they can also be hydrolysed to liberate the biologically active oestrogen moiety.

At least 50% of injected oestradiol and oestrone find their way into bile. Only 20–25% of oestriol follows that route, which is why conjugated oestriol is excreted almost totally unchanged (Slaunwhite *et al.*, 1973). Soon after injection of oestradiol a host of metabolites, mostly conjugated and many of them still unidentified, appear in bile fluid. After entering the intestine they are hydrolysed, mainly by the bacterial flora (Aldercreutz *et al.*, 1977; Back *et al.*, 1981). Most of the oestrogen which is reabsorbed is the unconjugated form (Back *et al.*, 1981). It is either reconjugated locally in the gut mucosa and returned by portal vein blood to the liver to repeat the cycle or reconjugated in the liver itself; only a small amount escapes conjugation and joins the systemic circulation. Therefore, as in the case of bile salts, the entero-hepatic circulation minimizes the loss of oestrogen in faeces. For this reason, and because of its greater affinity for sex steroid–binding globulin (Burton and Westphal, 1972), oestradiol is cleared much more slowly than oestriol. It is not known whether ageing affects the entero-hepatic circulation of steroids, although extra-hepatic biliary obstruction in older women potentially increases the rate of urinary excretion of oestradiol.

The most active biotransformations of oestradiol are shown in Fig. 2.8. They are essentially oxidative, with oestrone being a key intermediary. There is competitive hydroxylation of the 5-carbon D ring and the aromatic A ring of the steroid nucleus (Fig. 2.8). Hydroxylation at C-16 leads to oestriol formation via 16α-hydroxyoestrone. Hydroxylation at C-2 results in 2-hydroxyoestrone, a major urinary metabolite, which is partially and specifically *o*-methylated to 2-methoxyoestrone or, to a smaller extent, reduced to 2-hydroxyoestradiol (Fishman, 1981). These catechol oestrogens are formed in the liver and at other sites, including the hypothalamus (Fishman and Norton, 1975). Their rate of formation is expected to fall at menopause as a consequence of less ovarian oestrogen, but

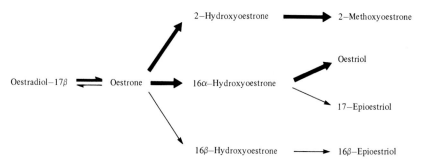

Fig. 2.8. Major pathways of metabolism of oestradiol in women. Thick arrows indicate predominant pathways.

concomitant changes in body composition could also affect the relative activity of alternative metabolic transformations (Fishman *et al.*, 1975). The oestrogenic activity of these substances is weak or non-existent, and they are remarkably evanescent. It has, therefore, been difficult to test whether they have a physiological role in gonadotrophin secretion or any involvement in the vasomotor disturbances of the climacteric (see Section 6.2).

After the menopause, representative values of metabolic clearance rates of oestradiol and oestrone fall by about 30% (Table 2.1). This order of change is similar to that of other steroids, which implies that common end organs, namely, the kidneys and liver, are at fault. Metabolic clearance rates may not change as abruptly at menopause as is indicated by Table 2.1; they may follow the steady downward trend of glomerular filtration rates during ageing (Goldman, 1977). Clearly, the reduced MCRs in older women tend to conserve any sex steroids present in the body.

3

The Follicular Store

3.1. Introduction

During the reproductive years, oestrogens are mainly produced by ovarian follicles and, in women and some animals, by their successors, the corpora lutea. Waves of follicular maturation are responsible for the hormonal manifestations of menstrual and oestrous cycles. Follicles are the developmental units of the ovary, each consisting of an oocyte enveloped by somatic cells. These cells are required for maintaining and controlling the development of the oocyte and, as described earlier, are the source of follicular oestradiol. This intimate relationship between germ cells and sex steroid–secreting cells contrasts with the situation in the testes, where their homologues are isolated from each other. Thus, ovarian oestrogen secretion falls when oocytes are depleted, whereas testosterone secretion continues from sterile testes. The biology of ovarian follicles must, therefore, be central to any discussion of the causes and timing of menopause. In the following sections the dynamic features of the follicular store are described and the age-related changes are discussed.

3.2. Formation of Oocytes and Follicles

In the late nineteenth century there was a lively debate on whether primordial germ cells are genuine progenitors of the definitive pool of the germ cells of later life. The school of Waldeyer (1870) claimed that they arise from proliferation of the epithelium covering the presumptive gonad, whereas Nussbaum (1880) stressed that a germ cell lineage is segregated from somatic cells at an early stage of embryogenesis. The second view was upheld by Weismann's (1885) theory of the continuity of germ plasm and is now well established.

Primordial germ cells of mammals are recognizable by their large size, low nuclear–cytoplasmic ratio and, in laboratory rodents and man, alkaline phosphatase activity at presomite and early somite stages. This enzyme is located in the Golgi apparatus and cell membrane, where it may be involved in the transport of metabolites. It is a useful marker for counting and tracing cells, and it enabled early workers to identify primordial germ cells in the yolk sac endoderm of 30-day-old human embryos (Witschi, 1948). It was assumed that germ cells originated from primary endoderm, but doubts arose when they were found at the base of the allantoic rudiment in mouse embryos. This finding implied a mesodermal origin in the primitive streak (Ożdzeński, 1967). More recently, elegant microsurgical techniques have provided new opportunities of studying the embryonic source of germ cells. Chimaerism among germ cells of mice could sometimes be identified following injection of epiblast cells into host blastocysts (Gardner and Rossant, 1976). Since epiblast and primary endoderm cells are already committed cell lines, it is concluded that germ cells are derived from epiblast which may subsequently migrate to the yolk sac.

Human primordial germ cells, estimated to number 1000–2000 by alkaline phosphatase activity, migrate to the gonadal ridge by active and passive movements, possibly guided by chemotaxis. Many cells are lost during transit, and only those reaching the favourable mesenchymal environment of the ridge will normally survive. Colonization of the gonadal anlagen by primordial germ cells is completed by 44–48 days after conception in man (12–14 days in mice) (Peters, 1970). By this time they have greatly multiplied in number. During the subsequent 5 months of gestation in man the germ cells can be seen in the

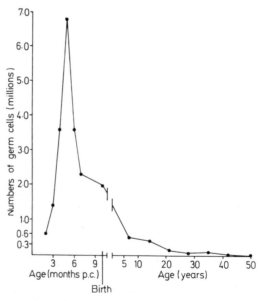

Fig. 3.1.   Variation in the total number of germ cells in human ovaries at prenatal and postnatal ages. [Reprinted with permission from T. G. Baker (1971), Radiosensitivity of mammalian oocytes with particular reference to the human female, *Am. J. Obstet. Gynecol.* **110**, 746–761.]

ingrowing "sex cords" of coelomic epithelium, where they reach a peak number of about 7 million (Baker, 1963) (Fig. 3.1). The germ cells may be unevenly distributed between the two ovaries, the imbalance being most marked in birds, where in many species the left ovary is the only functional gland. In some strains of mice (e.g. C57BL/6J) the number of follicles and ovulations is significantly greater in the right ovary, whereas, in women, there is tentative evidence of a left-sided bias in the number of primordial follicles (data of Block, 1952, re-analysed; $P < .05$). It is probable that unequal numbers of germ cells in adult ovaries reflect the number formed during oogenesis and that the more deficient organ will be the first one to fail during ageing.

Oogonia undergo a limited number of cell divisions and then enter meiosis, from which time they are known as "oocytes". Leptotene oocytes appear at about 4 months of gestation, and most oocytes become arrested at the diplotene stage 3 months later (Fig. 3.2). Some will not emerge from this "resting" phase until they are recruited for ovulation several decades later. In most species, including our own, oogonia do not persist after birth, and since oocytes are non-proliferating, a newborn infant already possesses its lifetime store.

In order to develop, oocytes require the physical and nutritional support of an envelope of somatic (follicle) cells, which also serve to regulate their develop-

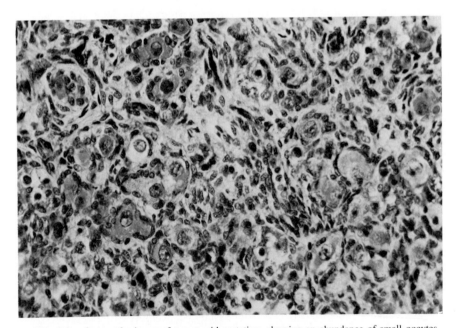

Fig. 3.2. Ovary of a human fetus at mid-gestation, showing an abundance of small oocytes, many of which have already reached diplotene of meiosis. Haematoxylin and eosin (X320).

ment. Follicle formation is a protracted process commencing at 5–6 months of gestation, with a few naked oocytes remaining for several months postpartum. Progenitors of granulosa follicle cells are derived, at least partly, from the embryonic mesonephros (Byskov, 1975). This system of tubules, known as the "rete ovarii", communicates with the ingrowing sex cords of ovarian epithelium. The prototype follicle consists of a single layer of pregranulosa cells. These "primordial" follicles are ovarian storehouses for oocytes. When oocytes are absent from the fetal gonad, the organ remains a small and undifferentiated "streak" which is incapable of producing steroid hormones in quantity. Sex steroids and gonadotrophins are probably not required for these early developments in the ovary (Baker and Neal, 1974), although they have dominating effects on follicles at later stages.

3.3. Initiation and Maintenance of Follicular Growth

Initiation of follicle growth is first recognised when the somatic cells increase in number and change from squamous to cuboidal forms. At the same time, oocytes enlarge and increase their production of RNA (Lintern-Moore and Moore, 1979), and mesenchymal cells in the stroma form a wreath around the small follicle. The latter cells will differentiate later into the inner secretory and external fibrous layers of the theca. Follicles leave the store of primordial stages at all ages and independently of the physiological state of the organism (e.g. pregnancy and lactation). Virtually nothing is known about the mechanism that activates them. Since they are recruited at a constant rate, it has been suggested that their activity is triggered by some stochastic event within the oocyte. However, few biological processes are truly random, and growth initiation is likely to depend on interactions between germ and somatic cells. There is some doubt whether gonadotrophins are required at this early stage of development. In adult ovaries of hypophysectomized mice, follicles grow to large multilaminar stages in the absence of these hormones (Jones and Krohn, 1961b). On the other hand, follicle growth in neonatal mice is inhibited by administering antiserum to gonadotrophins (Eshkol et al., 1971), and follicles fail to grow in anencephalic human fetuses in which pituitary function is also impeded (Baker and Scrimgeour, 1980). Whilst gonadotrophins may be required for the commencement of follicle growth in fetal or neonatal ovaries, most evidence suggests they are required mainly for larger follicles in postnatal life.

After its commencement, follicle growth continues without interruption until preovulatory maturation, unless atresia intervenes. The human primordial follicle measures 0.1 mm in diameter and contains approximately 10 pregranulosa cells, but when mature it measures >20 mm and contains 60 million granulosa cells (Gougeon, 1982). By this stage it has accumulated pools of extra-cellular fluid which coalesce to form an antrum. The follicle is called "Graafian" at this stage. In mice, primordial follicles are only slightly smaller than in women, but they form Graafian structures less than 1 mm in diameter, comprising only 50,000 cells. Stages of follicle growth are defined either by the number of granulosa cells or, more readily, by the number of cell layers (Figs. 3.3, 3.4).

Follicle growth is a lengthy process extending throughout several ovarian cycles. Unilaminar follicles in mice take at least 19 days to reach preovulatory size (Pedersen, 1970). In women, the corresponding period is probably greater than 3 months (Gougeon, 1982). Throughout adult life, murine follicles maintain a steady rate of growth which does not fall in middle age when ovulatory cycles cease (Faddy *et al.*, 1983; Gosden *et al.*, 1983b). Although comparable data

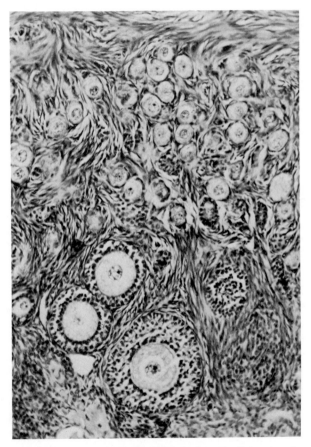

Fig. 3.3. Ovarian cortex of a young adult rhesus monkey, showing many primordial follicles, with follicular growth initiated at the inner boundary. Haematoxylin and eosin (X160).

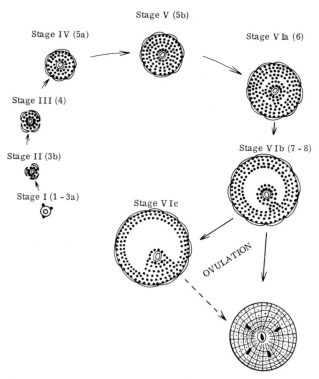

Fig. 3.4. Classification of follicle stages for the mouse ovary according to Mandl and Zuckerman (1951) (in roman numerals) and Pedersen and Peters (1968) (in arabic numerals). Primordial follicles (stage I/1–3a) grow through successive stages to antral (Graafian) size (stage VI/6–8) to ovulate and reorganize into corpora lutea or, in the absence of an ovulatory stimulus, enlarge to form follicular cysts (stage VIc). Follicles also terminate development in atresia at earlier stages, especially stages I, V and VIa.

cannot be obtained for human ovaries, gradual shortening of the follicular phase by 2–3 days over the menstrual lifespan (Vollman, 1977) would suggest that the velocity of growth of dominant follicles is increased unless ovulation occurs prematurely. A subtle, continuous change in the rate of growth can be attributed to corresponding changes in the pulsatile release of gonadotrophins, though this is a purely hypothetical suggestion and will be difficult to test (p. 89).

During the growth of follicle cells, their secretory activity and trophic requirements become differentiated. Granulosa cells possess receptors for many peptide and polypeptide hormones (FSH, LH, prolactin, growth hormone, LH releasing hormone and epidermal growth factor in rats), steroids (oestrogens, progesterone, glucocorticoids and testosterone), prostaglandins and even adrenergic agents. For normal maturation, they require a combination of extra- and intra-ovarian factors at specific stages in development. A fine balance between opposing stimulatory and inhibitory factors determines the fate of the follicle, whether it goes on to preovulatory maturation or atresia. One aspect of this balance is illustrated in patients with polycystic ovarian disease (Stein-Leventhal syndrome), in whom low levels of FSH combined with large pulses of plasma LH prevent follicles from developing beyond small antral stages which secrete androgens (Giorgi, 1963; Yen, 1980). Production of oestrogen can be restored by giving supplementary FSH (Erickson *et al.*, 1979). The failure of growing follicles to thrive in postmenopausal ovaries could be due to an inappropriate level or balance of gonadotrophic stimulation (Costoff and Mahesh, 1975). After the menopause, circulating levels of gonadotrophins rise steeply, with FSH becoming the more abundant of the two (see Section 4.4). Experimental studies have shown that excessive amounts of these hormones can suppress follicle cell growth (Rao *et al.*, 1978), oestrogen secretion (Moor, 1974) and even ovulation (Friedrich *et al.*, 1975). In contrast to the situation in women, rodents entering the anovulatory phase of life do not show the same elevation of gonadotrophin levels (Lu *et al.*, 1979) and have a normal succession of follicle stages which terminate in atresia after Graafian follicle maturity has been attained (Gosden *et al.*, 1983b).

3.4. Follicular Involution (Atresia)

Fewer than 0.01% of oocytes in women and 10% of oocytes in mice are ovulated. The remainder degenerate at various stages of follicular development at pre- and postnatal ages. Follicles undergoing degeneration are generally called ''atretic'', implying closure of the antrum (Gk. *a,* not; *tretos,* perforated). Small and medium-sized follicles are described in the same terms when moribund, even though neither of them possesses an antrum and different factors may be responsible for death. The greatest attrition of germ cells occurs prenatally during oogenesis. There are three waves of degeneration in human fetal ovaries involving (1) oogonia during mitosis (''atretic divisions''), (2) pachytene oocytes (''Z'' cells), and (3) diplotene oocytes. These reduce the number of germ cells from about 7 million to about 2 million at birth in both ovaries combined, and half of these are morphologically degenerate (Baker, 1963). Germ cells are also lost in fetal and neonatal rodent ovaries (Beaumont and Mandl, 1962). Small, non-growing follicles (stage I) die in large numbers between birth and puberty, with losses continuing throughout adult life in CBA mice (Faddy *et al.*, 1983). The death rate for human primordial follicles has not yet been estimated postnatally, though the data of Block (1952) would suggest that it is substantial.

Whereas preantral follicles at stages II–IV rarely appear degenerate, subsequent stages are highly vulnerable to atresia. Signs of atresia are normally seen first in the follicular epithelium and then in the theca and oocyte (Fig. 3.5). Apoptotic bodies, indicative of cell death, form in the mural population of

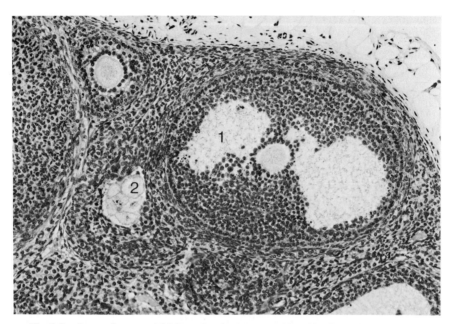

Fig. 3.5.   Ovary of a rat aged 25 days, showing two stages of atresia of large follicles. In (1) the oocyte is still intact, although there are many pycnotic cells in the granulosa layer. At a later stage (2) the antrum is obliterated and the oocyte is fragmented. Haematoxylin and eosin (X125).

granulosa cells; the follicular antrum shrinks and may contain exfoliated cells. These changes seem to alleviate the normal inhibitory effects of granulosa cells on the oocyte, which then resumes meiosis spontaneously and may undergo "pseudocleavage" divisions (Fig. 3.5). Theca cells may hypertrophy and even luteinize in some species. Advanced stages of atresia are reached in 3 days in mice (Byskov, 1974), but the process probably takes much longer in human ovaries, depending on follicle size. There may be vigorous infiltration of medium-sized human follicles by connective tissue to form avascular scars (corpora albicantia) which persist for long periods. When larger follicles become atretic, they may form cysts lined by fibrous, non-glandular cells. In ageing rodents, follicular cysts containing a clear or haemorrhagic fluid appear in small numbers in advance of the anovulatory phase of life, when they are more abundant (Peluso et al., 1979). These cysts are continuously being formed from smaller non-ovulatory follicles, but rapidly undergo atresia (Gosden et al., 1983b).

   Cell death occurs in many developing organs besides the ovary (e.g. muscle and spinal cord), but the mechanisms are likely to be organ specific. It has been suggested that cell death in the germ line is a consequence of a lethal load of mutations or errors of chromosome synapsis in some cells. There is, however, no experimental evidence that the bulk of germ cells are lost because of genetic faults. Moreover, oocyte death is not an inexorable process because the rate at which the follicular store is lost can be retarded in adult mice by hypophysectomy (Jones and Krohn, 1961b; Faddy *et al.*, 1983) and by long-term undernutrition (Nelson *et al.*, 1985) On the basis of hypophysectomy studies, Jones and Krohn (1959) postulated that the pituitary gland produces an atresia-promoting substance, but the effects of these treatments on oocytes are more likely to be nonspecific involving lowered cellular metabolism.

Graafian follicles evidently can be rescued from atresia. They can regenerate *in vitro* with healthy oocytes (Hay *et al.*, 1979) and are rescued *in vivo* by supplementary gonadotrophins (Peters *et al.*, 1975; Braw and Tsafriri, 1980b). There are two distinct types of atresia according to whether follicles fail to be selected for ovulation (small antral stages) or fail to be ovulated after having reached preovulatory maturity (larger stages). In the former case, FSH-sensitive aromatase is not activated/induced (McNatty *et al.*, 1979a), whereas, in the latter, follicles lose the aromatase activity they had acquired (Braw and Tsafriri, 1980a; Terranova, 1981). Large follicles are acutely dependent on gonadotrophic stimulation, and atresia follows abruptly after hypophysectomy (Braw *et al.*, 1981). The normal process of atresia could arise from understimulation because of lower plasma hormone levels or redistribution of ovarian blood. Whatever the mechanism, atresia leads to production of oestrogen, declining as production of progesterone rises (Braw and Tsafriri, 1980a; Terranova, 1981), whilst gonadotrophin receptors disappear (Carson *et al.*, 1979; Uilenbroek *et al.*, 1980). Follicle differentiation follows an alternative biosynthetic pathway if the normal steps towards ovulation are not taken, and this leads to reduced responsiveness to trophic stimuli and final limitation of the ability to be rescued.

3.5. Recruitment of Ovulatory Follicles

Many follicles begin to grow during each ovarian cycle, but few emerge as large, ovulable Graafian types. The number of these so-called dominant follicles is a species characteristic and is remarkably constant within individuals, despite variations in cycle length or size of the follicular store. The ovulation rate in animals (i.e. number of ova shed per cycle) is controlled by the global actions of gonadotrophins on the two ovaries. Local interactions between follicles seem unimportant because the distribution of ova shed by a pair of ovaries in polyovular species is binomial. Experimental support for a global mechanism has been provided by unilateral ovariectomy experiments, beginning with the historically important work of John Hunter (p. 115) and followed by many confirmatory studies of laboratory rodents. After surgery, the remaining ovary compensates for the loss of its partner by ovulating twice its normal quota of ova. This quota is maintained whilst sufficient stocks of follicles are available for recruitment, which is the greater proportion of normal cyclic life (Chatterjee and Greenwald, 1972; Brook *et al.*, 1984). Lipschutz (1927) used such findings in support of his "law of follicular constancy", but he drew the erroneous conclusion that the number of ovulatory follicles is regulated at the stage when they emerge from the non-growing store. Currently, it is thought that in rats, recruitment of the next set of preovulatory follicles is controlled by the surge of gonadotrophins that are associated with the dismissal of the present set by ovulation (Hirshfield and Midgley, 1978; Hoak and Schwartz, 1980). Thus, selection will take place among the population of small antral follicles, with the excess undergoing atresia.

In human ovaries, the ovulatory follicle is recruited from the population of antral stages at the end of the luteal phase preceding its ovulation (Baird, 1983). At this time there are about 6–30 antral follicles 1–15 mm in diameter in each ovary, but most of them, including all the large ones, are atretic (McNatty, 1982). Healthy antral follicles grow sluggishly, producing mainly androgens because plasma FSH levels are low during this phase (Fig. 3.6). Those that

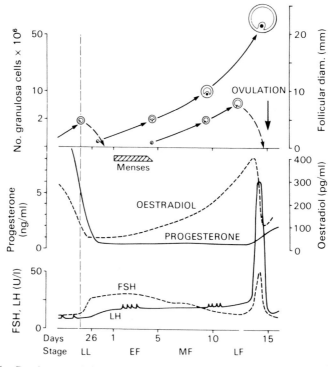

Fig. 3.6. Development of the human preovulatory follicle. Growth of antral follicles is suppressed during the luteal phase and recommences only when plasma levels of FSH and LH rise after luteal regression. EF, early follicular phase; MF, mid-follicular; LF, late follicular; EL, early luteal; ML, mid-luteal; LL, late luteal. The broken vertical line indicates the onset of luteal regression. (From Baird, 1983; reprinted with permission.)

develop FSH-sensitive aromatase activity in their granulosa cells will increase production of oestrogen and proceed towards ovulation. Only one or two such follicles exist *in toto* at the beginning of the follicular phase, others having become atretic. At present, it is not possible to predict which ones are selected. Further growth of healthy follicles depends on the significant elevation of plasma FSH levels at this time. These levels fall during the mid-follicular phase because of feedback effects of follicular oestrogen or the putative non-steroidal inhibitor, inhibin (de Jong and Sharpe, 1976). Since exogenous gonadotrophins given at this time have led to mutiple ovulations (Edwards *et al.*, 1972), it is likely that lower endogenous levels of FSH prevent recruitment of supernumerary follicles. Once selected, the dominant follicle seems to go through a "coasting" phase in which its growth is not impeded by lower FSH (Brown, 1978), perhaps because an extensive vascular net in its theca promotes the trapping of gonadotrophins (Zelesnik *et al.*, 1981).

There is clinical evidence to support the view that the number of follicles selected and the time of selection depend on a "window" of rising FSH secretion early in the cycle. Although ovarian responses to gonadotrophin therapy are highly variable in infertile women, a deviation in FSH levels of only 10% in a single individual may alter the number of ovulations (Brown, 1978). On the other hand, attempts to use plasma hormone profiles to predict ovulation rates in sheep have been disappointing, leading to the suspicion that FSH action is modulated by other factors (Scaramuzzi and Radford, 1983). In cynomolgus monkeys, removal of the corpus luteum resulted in early emergence of a new follicle in the opposite ovary in 90% of cases; hence, it has been suggested that gradients of progesterone determine which follicles are recruited (Goodman *et al.*, 1977; Goodman and Hodgen, 1979). At present, there is no such evidence of local effects in women (Nilsson *et al.*, 1982), although the search for modulating factors will continue. Recently, it was reported that human follicular fluid contains proteins that interfere with responses to gonadotrophins (DiZerega *et al.*, 1983), but it is not known whether these proteins are involved physiologically in the selection of dominant follicles.

The number of ovulatory follicles selected during a cycle is affected by ageing. The incidence of dizygotic (but not monozygotic) twins increases with maternal age until about age 37 (Fig. 3.7). This increase is presumed to parallel the incidence of binovular cycles rather than reflect greater fetal survival *in utero*. A rising incidence of binovular cycles seems to proceed *pari passu* with shorter follicular phase length, and both might be explained by a rising output of pituitary FSH. This explanation is supported by the established dose relationship between FSH and ovulation rate, though there are few reports that FSH rises in normal women before the fifth decade (Reyes *et al.*, 1977). The alternative explanations that binovular follicles are more common or that follicles are more responsive to FSH during ageing seem improbable.

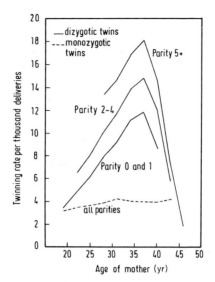

Fig. 3.7. Monozygotic and dizygotic twinning rates in women according to age and parity (Italian data, 1949–1954). (From Bulmer, 1970; reprinted with permission.)

Parity has less effect than age on the incidence of dizygotic twins (Fig. 3.7), though this too could be explained by FSH action. An effect of parity on ovulation rate is found in animals. The steadily rising number of pups born to mice during the first few litters is attributed to more ovulations rather than less prenatal mortality (MacDowell and Lord, 1925; Kennedy and Kennedy, 1972). The rise in body weight or the change in body composition of the mother resulting from earlier pregnancies could be important factors. For instance, expansion of the distribution volume for hormones might decrease feedback actions of gonadal hormones, or subtle changes in metabolic activity might affect neurosecretion or hormone action. Whilst these mechanisms are entirely conjectural, the phenomenon of ''flushing'' in sheep is concrete evidence of a link between energy balance/stores and ovarian function (Rattray, 1977). Increased caloric intake during the preovulatory period leads to 10–20% more ovulations per cycle provided that animals are prevented from becoming fat during summer months.

The steeply declining rate of dizygotic twins from age 37 occurs at a time when circulating amounts of FSH are, if anything, rising. This may be explained partly by increased fetal mortality among twin pregnancies of older women or by the waning fertility of the father, but waning ovarian function is likely to be more important. In twin-prone women, declining numbers of follicles available for recruitment will finally limit double ovulations (Bulmer, 1970) and may even bring about earlier menopause (James, 1979). That exceptionally fecund women should cease reproduction earlier may seem paradoxical, but data in rats show the number of ovulations is inversely related to the size of the follicular store (Land *et al.*, 1974).

3.6. Follicular Dynamics throughout Life

The major characteristics of ovarian follicular dynamics have been stated already, namely, establishment by the time of birth of a large store of nongrowing follicles from which recruits are drawn at a constant rate into the growing follicle population. This population, in turn, supplies recruits for ovulation, and surplus follicles are eliminated by atresia. The fixed rate at which follicles are initiated into growth helps to account for demographic data which show that the age of menopause is relatively independent of a wide range of physiological and environmental factors, apart from those that actually destroy follicles (see Section 1.5).

The rates of follicle utilization and atresia have been studied in greatest detail in rodents. Two methods have been used. In the first, proliferating granulosa cells are labelled during the S-phase of the cell cycle with tritiated thymidine and analysed by autoradiography (Fig. 3.8). The rates of transit between successive

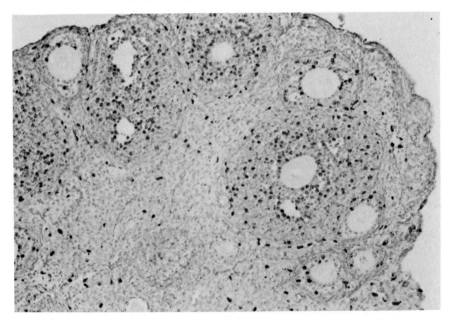

Fig. 3.8. Autoradiograph of an adult mouse ovary 1 hr after injecting tritiated thymidine. All multilaminar follicles are labelled by silver grains which indicate that follicle growth, once initiated, is continuous without interruption until the follicles either ovulate or become atretic. Haemalum and eosin (X125).

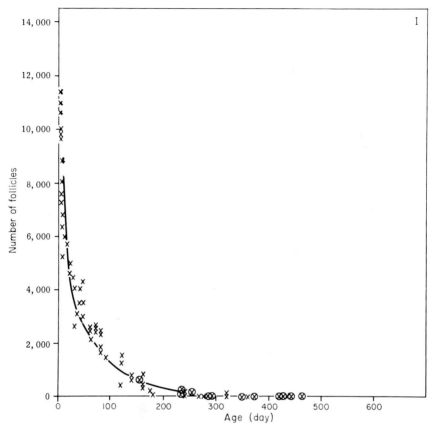

Fig. 3.9. Variations in the number of follicles of differing sizes (stages I–V+) in non-pregnant CBA mice between birth and senility. Data for virgin (x) and ex-breeder mice (⊗) are presented. Means ± SE have been estimated using a mathematical model. (From Faddy *et al.*, 1983; originally published in the *J. Endocrinol.*)

follicle stages can then be estimated from measurements of granulosa cell numbers and cell cycle time because once growth has been initiated there is no further resting stage (Pedersen, 1970). In the second method, the number of follicles at each stage of development (I–VI) is counted in histological sections. Rates of follicle growth and atresia can then be estimated at all ages using a mathematical model (Faddy *et al.*, 1976). Data obtained by Jones and Krohn (1961a) have been fitted to this model (see Fig. 3.9 and Table 3.1 with Fig. 3.4 for the classification of follicle stages). At birth, about 9400 stage I (primordial) follicles are present in a pair of ovaries, no other stages being present yet (Faddy *et al.*, 1983). Soon afterwards, a proportion of these follicles begins to move

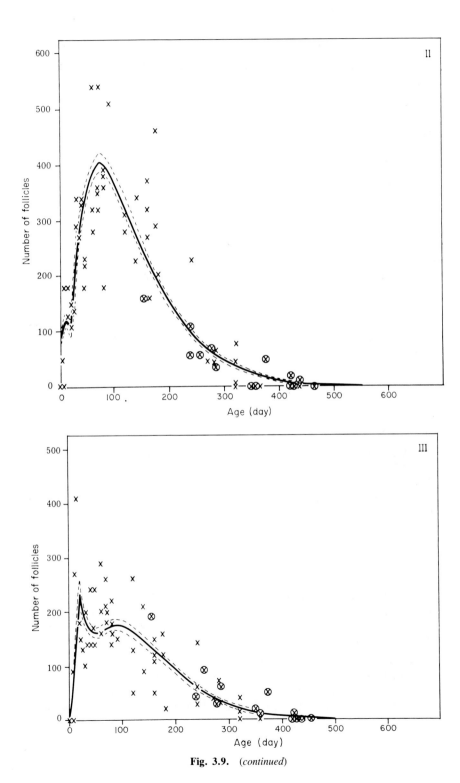

Fig. 3.9. (*continued*)

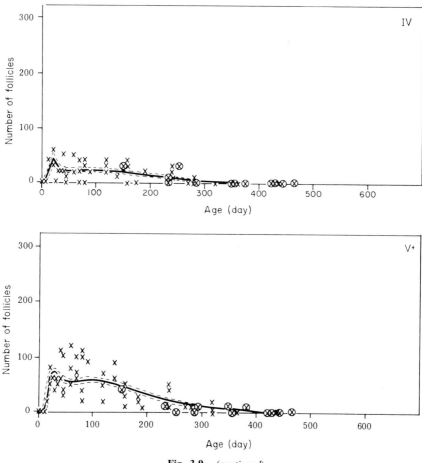

Fig. 3.9. (*continued*)

through successive stages of development. The number present in each category is determined by stage- and age-specific growth and death rates in the precursor pool and are described by Poisson statistics (Table 3.1). More than half of the original stock of follicles is lost during the first 20 days of life. Since fewer than 10% of those leaving the non-growing store (437 our of 5059) reach stage II, more than 90% must have died. Differences between the number of follicles leaving and entering successive stages (see columns) are small (Table 3.1). Most of those reaching stage II proceed to become large preantral and antral follicles (V+), although they fail to mature and ovulate at prepubertal ages. The high death rate among small follicles before puberty (<5 weeks) prevents an explosive increase in the number of follicles in the growing population. After-

TABLE 3.1

Mean Number of Follicles (from the Fitted Model) in CBA Mouse Ovaries Leaving and Entering Five Groups (Primordial to Graafian) at Specified Ages throughout Life[a]

Age span (days)	Movement of follicles from and to successive groups								
	I→	→II	II→	→III	III→	→IV	IV→	→V+	V+→
0–20	5058.9	437.3	334.0	334.0	97.5	97.5	51.6	51.6	0.0
20–30	597.8	155.2	31.7	31.7	84.6	84.6	103.0	103.0	83.5
30–60	1341.5	348.4	185.1	185.1	203.6	203.6	208.8	208.8	255.3
60–90	858.5	222.9	223.9	223.9	212.1	212.1	210.4	210.4	207.4
90–120	549.3	142.6	203.3	203.3	213.6	213.6	214.6	214.6	215.2
120–150	351.5	91.3	164.3	164.3	190.1	190.1	193.5	193.5	200.4
150–180	224.9	58.4	124.6	124.6	154.7	154.7	158.8	158.8	168.5
180–210	143.9	37.4	90.8	90.8	118.7	118.7	122.5	122.5	132.1
210–240	92.1	23.9	64.4	64.4	87.3	87.3	90.5	90.5	98.7
240–270	58.9	15.3	44.8	44.8	62.4	62.4	64.9	64.9	71.4
270–300	37.7	9.8	30.7	30.7	43.7	43.7	45.5	45.5	50.4
300–330	24.1	6.3	20.8	20.8	30.1	30.1	31.4	31.4	34.9
330–360	15.4	4.0	14.0	14.0	20.5	20.5	21.4	21.4	23.9
360–390	9.9	2.6	9.3	9.3	13.8	13.8	14.4	14.4	16.1
390–420	6.3	1.6	6.2	6.2	9.2	9.2	9.7	9.7	10.9
420–450	4.0	1.1	4.1	4.1	6.1	6.1	6.4	6.4	7.2
450–480	2.6	0.7	2.7	2.7	4.1	4.1	4.3	4.3	4.8
480–510	1.7	0.4	1.8	1.8	2.7	2.7	2.8	2.8	3.2

[a] From M. J. Faddy, R. G. Gosden and R. G. Edwards, unpublished.

wards, the death rate falls to produce the characteristic biphasic distribution of follicles of different stages (Fig. 3.9). In the CBA strain, continuing death in the primordial stages is responsible for the loss of more follicles from the store at all ages than are accounted for by those initiating growth. This explains why the ovary is depleted of oocytes at little more than 1 year of age, with early disappearance of ovarian cycles at 10–11 months. Since small follicles are lost continuously throughout life, all animals will eventually become sterile if their survival is prolonged. Therefore it is not surprising that neither pregnancy (Fig. 3.9) nor unilateral ovariectomy (Baker et al., 1980) has much effect on the number of small follicles remaining at advanced ages.

Far more follicles enter the growing population at most ages than are required for ovulation. In CBA mice, the number of follicles at each stage of growth reaches peak values during adult life at about 100 days (Fig. 3.9). These enable the ovary to superovulate when stimulated by supplementary gonadotrophins following removal of the contralateral ovary or treatment with exogenous gonadotrophins. The subsequent decline in the number of growing follicles is a reflection of fewer being recruited from a dwindling store. Only 21 follicles entered the preovulatory stages V and VI at 330–360 days of age, whereas there were 10 times as many at ages 60–90 days (Table 3.1). Thus, the ability of the ovary to superovulate is expected to fall steadily during ageing, and this has been confirmed experimentally (Beatty, 1958; R. G. Gosden, unpublished). Unfortunately, present mathematical models cannot provide precise estimates of the dynamics of antral follicles because these follicles are fewer in number and fluctuate during the cycle. The number attaining preovulatory maturity is maintained in CBA mice until 300 days of age, when the natural ovulation rate begins to fall. The ability to sustain or increase the ovulation rate appears to depend on a reduction in the proportionate incidence of atresia in medium-sized follicles rather than on the recruitment of more follicles from the store (Gosden *et al.*, 1983a).

Few workers have attempted a differential count of the number of follicles in adult human ovaries, the only substantial data having been obtained from cadavers by Block (1952). The reasons for the limited information on this important subject are plain. Premenopausal ovaries (if obtainable) can yield 2000 paraffin sections of 10-μm thickness, requiring weeks of laborious microscopy to obtain reliable follicle counts in just one ovary. Despite limitations of the data (viz. sampling every 200th section and no estimates of atresia), Block's work seems to establish that numbers of primordial follicles fall continuously during adult life (Fig. 3.1). Their distribution by age would be expected to be an exponential or double exponential, as in rodents, but closer inspection of the data shows that a quadratic function provides a marginally better fit for human primordial follicles ($P = .065$). In view of the limited data, this conclusion must be tentative but, if confirmed, would establish that these follicles are lost at an increasing rate during ageing.

Despite the sampling errors which occur in most quantitative studies of the follicular population, the remarkable variations in primordial follicle numbers in individuals of the same age probably reflect real differences. Since the numbers at a given stage and age can vary as much as twofold in syngeneic mice (Fig. 3.9), biological differences have environmental causes, and these are likely to operate prenatally during oogenesis. Such variation in data adds further uncertainty to the already hazardous procedure of extrapolation. Nevertheless, if Block's data are extrapolated to the median age of menopause of 50 in contemporary Swedes (Table 1.2), only a few hundreds or thousands of primordial follicles evidently remain. This suggests that primary ovarian failure causes the final cessation of menses in mid-life and the inability of postmenopausal ovaries to respond to gonadotrophins. Irregular menstrual cycles preceding the menopause can be attributed to irregular recruitment of multilaminar follicles, which decline in number in the fifth decade of life (Block, 1952). However, only after the majority of small follicles have been lost (at about 36 years of age) does the menstrual cycle become most stable and regular (Treloar *et al.*, 1967; Vollman, 1977; Fig. 3.10). Thus, age-related variations in the timing of the cycle probably depend to some extent on factors which are independent of the diminishing follicular store.

3.7. Precocious Ovarian Failure (Precocious Menopause)

Primary, irreversible ovarian failure occurs before middle age in some individuals, but the biological effects are essentially independent of age, except in

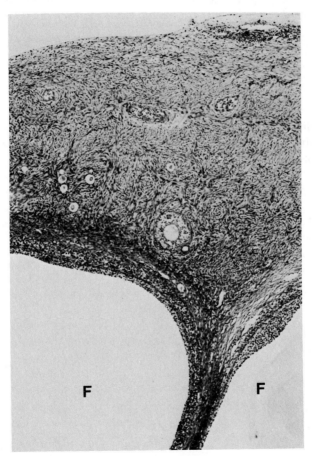

Fig. 3.10.   Representative section of the ovarian cortex of a 34-year-old woman, showing that small follicles are sparse by this age. Graafian stages (F) are present. Haematoxylin and eosin (X50).

children, in whom there are additional effects on adolescent growth and maturation. This condition is diagnosed when acyclic women have plasma levels of FSH exceeding 40–50 mIU/ml, a sign of an inactive negative feedback pathway from the ovary (Goldenberg *et al.*, 1973). This shibboleth is not, however, entirely reliable and the possibility of pregnancy should not be ruled out (Rebar *et al.*, 1982). The limitations of present definitions could be overcome if more stringent criteria were adopted (e.g. by extending the duration of amenorrhoea), but this would be at the expense of lost time in providing hormone replacement therapy. The best criterion of menopause would be complete absence of ovarian follicles in serial histological sections, but quantitative studies of this kind are impractical on a routine basis and biopsy material is not always available (see Section 3.6).

The follicular store may become depleted at any age after it is formed. There is, however, no agreed-on lower normal age limit for the menopause, and so widely differing and arbitrary limits have been used, ranging from 30 to 45 years. This unsatisfactory state of affairs is likely to continue because of the difficulties of estimating menopausal age in the normal population (see Section 1.5). Thus, there are no reliable estimates of the frequency of precocious menopause in any population. Even if data became available, they could not be applied universally; if they could, by Western standards, many poor women in parts of the developing world might be described as having precocious menopause.

Cases of precocious menopause can be divided into two categories according to whether or not substantial numbers of follicles remain. In many cases, there is evidence that ovaries are afollicular, and a number of factors can account for this condition.

Genetic Factors. A substantial proportion of all women presenting with precocious ovarian failure have an abnormal karyotype, hence the term "chromosomally incompetent ovarian failure" (Tho and McDonough, 1982). The most familiar cases of ovarian dysgenesis occur among women with X-chromosome monosomy (Turner's syndrome) or XX/XO mosaicism. The histological appearance of ovaries in these individuals suggests that a primordial germ cell population is established but fails to thrive. The timing of the loss of germ cells is highly variable. Anovular streak gonads are common at pre- and postnatal ages among XO individuals (Carr *et al.*, 1968), but some ovaries have a population of oocytes of normal appearance at full term which, in rare cases, provide an opportunity for pregnancy before an early menopause (Reyes *et al.*, 1976; King *et al.*, 1978). Oogonia and oocytes might fail to thrive either because of the generalized debility of some fetuses or because of gene dosage effects. Unlike somatic cells, in which only one member of each pair of X chromosomes is genetically active, both sex chromosomes of 46,XX fetal oocytes are normally active (Gartler *et al.*, 1973) following reactivation shortly before meiosis (Monk and McLaren, 1981). Since single chromosomes do not compensate for the loss of their opposite number, there is a deficiency of gene products in oocytes of XO fetuses. Further progress in this field might be gained by the study of XO mice for, although they are more fertile than XO women, they too have fewer oocytes than do normal siblings, and consequently their reproductive lifespan closes prematurely (Lyon and Hawker, 1973; Burgoyne and Baker, 1981a). Apart from runts, XO mouse fetuses establish normal numbers of germ cells and the deficiencies of postnatal life have been traced to an excess of "Z" cells at the end of gestation (Burgoyne and Baker, 1981b).

Trisomy affects the follicle reserve in different ways depending on whether sex chromosomes or autosomes are involved. Most women presenting the X chromosome in triplicate have normal phenotype and fertility, although ovarian failure occurs early in a few of them (Villanueva and Rebar, 1983). In contrast, trisomies of chromosomes 18 (Edward's syndrome) and 21 (Down's syndrome) are associated with reduced numbers of both non-growing and growing follicles (Russell and Altschuler, 1975; Højager *et al.*, 1978). Other types of autosomal trisomy probably effect gonadal development, but such fetuses are not viable anyway.

Most cases of streak gonads occur sporadically in the population but familial transmission is seen in a number of rare conditions, especially 46,XY and 46,XX gonadal dysgenesis (German *et al.*, 1978; Simpson, 1983). It is difficult to establish whether specific genes cause precocious ovarian failure because opportunities for studying them are rare and there are additional practical and ethical constraints. However, on the basis of a few favourable pedigrees it has been possible to obtain evidence that premature ovarian failure can be heritable, transmission occurring via either maternal or paternal relatives and probably involving an autosomal dominant factor (Mattison *et al.*, 1984). In mice, heritable factors clearly influence the size and rate of utilization of the follicular store, though differences between inbred strains almost certainly have a polygenic basis (Jones and Krohn, 1961a). Some gene mutations in mice having pleiotrophic effects cause ovarian dysgenesis. In the Steel mutant (*SL*) a streak gonad forms when primordial germ cells fail to proliferate (McCoshen, 1982), and mutant alleles of the *W* series are generally associated with germ cell hypoplasia and sterility (Mintz and Russell, 1957; Murphy, 1972).

Immunological Factors. Autoimmune phenomena may lead to premature sterility in rodents as a result of total destruction of germ cells. Such damage occurs when neonatal mice are thymectomized (Michael *et al.*, 1981; Nishizuka *et al.*, 1981), which may explain why mutant mice (*nu,nu*), which are congenitally deficient in T cells, are relatively infertile. It is interesting that ovarian hypoplasia also occurs in children with ataxia telangiectasia in whom thymus tissue is also deficient or absent (Miller and Chatten, 1967).

A substantial proportion of women having premature menopause possess circulating anti-ovarian antibodies though signs of infiltration of the ovary by mononuclear cells is required to establish the presence of autoimmune destructive activity (Coulam and Ryan, 1979). In some cases, evidence of such damage coexists with autoimmune disease involving other endocrine glands with clinical expressions of Addison's disease, hypoparathyroidism and Hashimoto's thyroiditis (de Moraes-Ruehsen *et al.*, 1972; Vasquez and Kenny, 1973). The aetiology of this complex of diseases is poorly understood. Autosensitization to common antigens expressed on cell surfaces may explain why several glands are involved simultaneously, although T cell function might also be impaired (Mathur *et al.*, 1980a). Sometimes chronic yeast infections of the lower genital tract (*Candida* sp.) lead to menstrual irregularity and even ovarian failure, apparently as a consequence of autoimmune damage (Mathur *et al.*, 1980b). The combination of these problems can also be explained by common antigenic epitopes in ovarian cells and the microorganism.

Cytotoxic Drugs. Clinical use of drugs in the treatment of cancer, rheumatoid arthritis and other serious diseases frequently leads to temporary cessation of menses. If treatment is prolonged, destruction of follicles may result in earlier menopause (Rose and Davis, 1977). These effects are obviously more important for young women and children than for the majority of patients at risk, who are much older (Warne *et al.*, 1973; Himelstein-Braw *et al.*, 1977, 1978). Damage can be inflicted inadvertently on the fetal gonad since alkylating agents such as busulphan are transmitted across the placenta following maternal administration (Diamond *et al.*, 1960). Damage to proliferating primordial germ cells may be significant later in life because they have only a limited ability to undergo compensatory growth after withdrawal of treatment (Tam and Snow, 1981), and destruction of germ cells after oogenesis is serious because they are irreplaceable.

Ionizing Radiations. Extensive studies have been made of the cellular and genetic effects on the ovary of X and γ rays because these can penetrate deeply into tissues. Cell-killing activity varies with age, species and the manner of administration (single dose or fractionated). In rodent fetuses, the oogonial stage is the most radio-sensitive of all stages in oogenesis, although sensitivity rises again in early dictyotene when follicles are forming. Primordial follicles in rats and mice are among the most sensitive groups of cells. Fortunately, those of monkeys and women are far less vulnerable to irradiation, probably because of differing chromosome configurations and metabolism (Baker, 1971; Baker and Neal, 1977). Multi-layered follicles of all species studied so far are vulnerable to irradiation because of their mitotic activity. Therapeutic exposure of the pelvic region in women can lead to amenorrhoea, but this is usually temporary if the dose is <400 R (fractionated). The outcome will vary according to age, with the probability of resuming cycles after treatment falling in older women.

Low-energy radiation is of little biological significance unless the isotope is actually incorporated into ovarian cells. Tritiated nucleosides are especially haz-ardous for proliferating germ cells since most of the energy is dissipated within the nucleus (Baker and McLaren, 1973).

Other Disease Effects. Irreversible damage of the ovary during the course of disease is usually iatrogenic, although there are minor exceptions. Some infil-trative diseases (e.g. tuberculosis) have serious effects on the genital tract with involvement of the ovary, but permanent loss of ovulatory function is rare. Viral diseases (e.g. mumps) can cause oophoritis, which may be a more extensive problem than rare case reports would suggest (Morrison *et al.*, 1975).

Non-infectious diseases, in addition to those mentioned above in the context of genetics and immunology, have profound effects on fecundity. Where there is a deficiency of 17α-hydroxylase, androgen and oestrogen production falls and pregnenolone and progesterone are metabolized by an alternative pathway, lead-ing to excess production of mineralocorticoids. This rare disease presents symp-toms of sexual immaturity and primary amenorrhoea, with castrate levels of gonadotrophins and oestrogen (Goldsmith *et al.*, 1967). Ovarian failure is there-fore due to a lack of oestrogen and a consequent inability of follicles to grow rather than to early depletion of the follicular store. Hence, these ovaries resem-ble more closely those of individuals with hypopituitarism or with the so-called resistant ovary syndrome, in which follicles are unresponsive to FSH (Jones and de Moraes-Ruehsen, 1969). On the other hand, precocious menopause caused by the congenital disorder of metabolism, galactosaemia, (Kaufman *et al.*, 1981) may be due to formation of a smaller follicular store because galactose or its metabolites have toxic effects on germ cells in the developing ovary of animal models (Chen *et al.*, 1981). This would explain why early menstrual failure is not overcome by feeding patients a galactose-restricted diet from infancy. Possi-ble effects of inadequate diets on the age of menopause in normal women have been discussed elsewhere (see Section 1.5).

Blindness is thought to advance the timing of menarche, and there is now tentative evidence that it also leads to later menopause (Lehrer, 1981). Such results have been attributed to the activity of the pineal gland, which is affected by photoperiod, but there is little physiological evidence at present to support the claim that it affects the length of menstrual life.

Alcoholism. Chronic alcoholism has complex effects on nutrition and metab-olism. It causes hypogonadism and infertility in both sexes (van Thiel and

Lester, 1976), but it is not known whether gonadal injury is permanent or reversible, and practical difficulties of working with alcoholic patients hamper further study. In adult rats, ethanol inhibits follicular growth and luteinization (van Thiel *et al.*, 1978), but it remains unknown whether the size of the non-growing store of follicles is reduced. Of greater concern is the unanswered question of whether alcohol consumed during pregnancy causes lasting damage to the fetal gonad.

Partial Ovariectomy (Oophorectomy). Since oocytes cannot be replaced after birth, removal of any ovarian tissue potentially reduces the remaining period of fecundity. It has been postulated that the dynamics of ovarian follicle growth initiation are stochastic. This would imply that substantial amounts of tissue would have to be lost in order to cause an obvious advance of menopausal age, and this can be illustrated by a simple example. If it is assumed that the normal age for complete depletion of ovarian follicles in a woman is 60 years, then hemi-ovariectomy at birth would advance the time by 30 years according to a linear model of follicle utilization, but by only 5 years according to an exponential model. This hypothesis has not been verified in any primate species, but supporting evidence is provided by longitudinal studies of unilaterally ovariectomized CBA mice (Brook *et al.*, 1984). Removal of one ovary at 50 days of age resulted in complete cessation of cycles by 330 days in half the population, whereas this point was reached 40 days later in controls with both ovaries present.

The dynamics of follicle utilization would also serve to minimize differences in menopausal age, despite considerable natural variation in the size of the follicle population. Nevertheless, the present policy of conserving healthy ovaries during gynaecological surgery should not be relaxed since even a small advance in age of menopause is usually undesirable.

3.8. Anatomy of the Postmenopausal Ovary

Follicular deficiency is the most striking morphological feature of the human ovary after menopause and has profound importance for ovarian physiology and pathology. As mentioned earlier, the ovary is not completely afollicular at the time of menopause, although it may eventually reach this state. The postmenopausal ovary is composed mainly of "stroma", which is a collective term for supporting (connective tissue) cells, contractile cells and interstitial cells. The interstitium is widely thought to be derived from theca cells that return to the stromal population after follicular atresia. Besides stroma, the only other bulky materials in postmenopausal ovaries are large fibrous bodies which are relics of corpora lutea of the final menstrual years (Fig. 3.11). The walls of

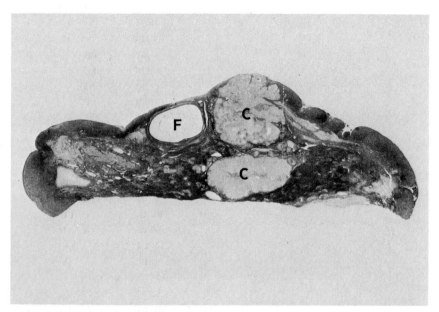

Fig. 3.11. Perimenopausal human ovary (age 51 years), showing abundant stromal tissue and two corpora albicantia (C). One cystic (atretic ?) follicle (F) is present. There are no small follicles in this section. Haematoxylin and eosin (X5.5).

ovarian arteries, as elsewhere in the genital tract, become thicker and calcified during ageing, particularly in multiparous women (Fig. 3.12). In middle age, there is surface folding of the organ because atrophic changes within are not matched by corresponding dynamic changes of the ovarian epithelium. Later, the ovary shrinks to a small, pigmented structure, but is not entirely without endocrine activity (see Section 2.3).

There is a striking contrast of appearance between ovaries of postmenopausal women and aged sub-human primates on the one hand and those of acyclic rodents of middle age on the other. Apart from some mutants and inbred strains, most rodents still possess some ovarian follicles in extreme old age. At this time the rodent ovary is dominated by interstitial tissue and Graafian follicles, which undergo cystic enlargement (''overripening'') rather than ovulation (Fig. 3.13). In later life, long after fertility is lost, these follicles may ovulate and luteinize to form functional corpora lutea of pseudopregnancy (p. 71). Rodent ovaries do not accumulate large residual fibrous structures, nor do their blood vessels undergo the same degree of sclerosis as in primates. Their interstitium may contain cells in which nuclear chromatin is arranged radially (''wheel cells''). Although this condition needs re-evaluation in the light of recent hormone assays, these cells have been interpreted as evidence of LH deficiency, since similar cells are seen

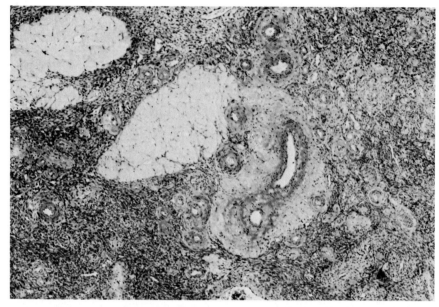

Fig. 3.12. Postmenopausal human ovary at low magnification. Blood vessel walls are sclerotic; stromal cells are abundant and interspersed with fibrous remnants of atretic follicles and corpora lutea. Haematoxylin and eosin (X50).

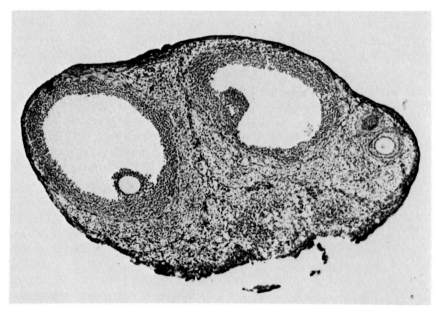

Fig. 3.13. Anovulatory ovary of a 16-month-old C57BL/6J mouse. There are few small or medium-sized follicles and no corpora lutea. Two cystic (anovulatory) follicles are present. Haematoxylin and eosin (X70).

in hypophysectomized animals and a normal pattern of chromatin can be restored by gonadotrophins (Crumeyrolle-Arias *et al.*, 1976). Other cells within the stroma contain abundant lipochrome pigments which are responsible for the yellow-brown hue of ageing rodent ovaries. These pigments, which are found in primate ovaries to a lesser extent, probably represent indigestible residues of autolysis and phagocytosis of follicular and luteal tissue.

Pathological changes in ageing ovaries depend less on chronological age than on the time when follicles are depleted. Such changes appear precociously when animal ovaries become sterile following neonatal thymectomy (Michael *et al.*, 1981) and ionizing irradiation (Peters, 1969), as well as in mutant and inbred strains characterized by early loss of oocytes (Murphy, 1972; Thung, 1961). These changes involve cellular proliferation as well as atrophy. Thung (1961) suggested that the former is due to hypergonadotrophism, but there are likely to be local contributing factors (e.g. rising androgen : oestrogen ratio) because pathological changes do not emerge evenly in the gland but begin at sites that are first depleted of follicles (unpublished observations). Stroma cell hyperplasia and hilus cell prominence in human ovaries are usually attributed to stimulation by postmenopausal levels of gonadotrophins (Sternberg, 1949). In mice, the surface epithelium grows inwards to mingle with the ovarian rete and form a complex internal structure of "testis-like" tubules, epithelial cords and "anovular follicles". A peculiar form of follicular atresia may give rise to similar structures in rats (Crumeyrolle-Arias and Aschheim, 1981). In primates, ovarian epithelia tend to proliferate for a relatively short period, and they tend to form papillary projections (Graham *et al.*, 1979). These differing patterns of proliferative activity in rodent and primate ovaries might therefore explain the higher frequency of tubular adenomata and granulosa cell tumours in the former group.

4

The Ovarian Clock

4.1. Early Concepts of the Menstrual Cycle

Periodic menstrual activity has fascinated humans since antiquity. Frequently it has acquired special cultural significance in religious ritual and superstition (Frazer, 1935; Lévi-Strauss, 1966). Among other notions, it was thought to be responsible for eliminating toxins accumulating in blood, which seemed to explain the associated pain, odour and appearance of the menstrual flow. This ancient view can be traced back to Hippocrates and was upheld subsequently by Aristotle, Galen and Pliny, remaining popular in Europe even into the nineteenth century. Early scientific speculation in the first half of that century was equally faulty. Too much attention was paid to the similarity in the length of the lunar cycle and the "typical" menstrual cycle (28 days). Indeed, the word "menses" is derived from this connection (L. *mensis:* month).

The first experimental evidence for a role of ovaries in the menstrual cycle is attributed to Percival Pott, a London surgeon, who reported that removal of both ovaries in a young woman for correction of "ovarian herniae" resulted in atrophy of her breasts and cessation of menstruation (Pott, 1775). Pott did not comment on the physiological significance of his findings, which went unrecognized for nearly 40 years. John B. Davidge, an American student of medicine in Edinburgh, learned of this case. His observation that loss of much larger quantities of blood by venesection than by menstruation did not interfere with menstrual flow led him to conclude that the latter "is attributable to a peculiar condition of the ovaries serving as a source of excitement to the vessels of the womb, rather than to the doctrine of repletion of the body" (Davidge, 1814). Despite this astute conclusion, the traditional views persisted for many years, and the ovary was not recognized as an organ of internal secretion until the end of the nineteenth century.

The foundations of present knowledge concerning the timing of ovulation and the cyclical fluctuations of ovarian hormones were laid in the 1930s, a golden decade of discoveries in reproductive physiology and biochemistry. Later, the neuroendocrine mechanisms controlling the cycle were studied in great detail in rats. Whilst information about primates was scarce, there was little reason to doubt the general validity of the rat model except, of course, for the peculiar phenomenon of menstruation itself. But recent research casts doubt on this assumption. Some background information on the differing physiological mechanisms is therefore essential before proceeding to describe and explain the effects of ageing on the ovarian cycles of women and animals.

4.2. Physiological Regulation of Ovarian Cycles

During the 1920s there was a growing appreciation of the importance of feedback mechanisms in physiology. Their greatest proponent was W. B. Cannon, who coined the term ''homeostasis'' and broadcast the new concepts in his influential book *The Wisdom of the Body* (1932). Reproductive biologists grasped the implications for their own field, and it was soon recognised that gonadal function might be controlled by feedback interactions with the pituitary gland (Moore and Price, 1932). At an early stage the hypothalamus was suspected to be a key structure in reproduction, containing a ''sex centre'' to mediate actions of sex steroids on the underlying pituitary gland (Hohlweg and Junkmann, 1932). During the subsequent 50 years, a major goal of reproduction research has been to elucidate the neuroendocrine control mechanisms and identify pathways of communication between the brain and gland. Luteinizing hormone-releasing hormone (LHRH, also known as GnRH) was isolated from hypothalamic extracts and characterized in 1971 (Matsuo *et al.*, 1971), the same year as Harris reviewed the early history of the field in the prestigious Dale Lecture (Harris, 1972). The neuropeptide LHRH is a key substance for reproduction because, as Harris had postulated much earlier, it is the signal by which information processed by the brain is passed to the pituitary gland.

A number of studies showed that the ovulatory surge of LH (and FSH) in rats is elicited by neural activity associated with the internal circadian rhythm. That a cerebral clock was responsible for timing ovulation was shown clearly by the inhibitory action of barbiturate administration during a ''critical period'' on the afternoon before oestrus (Everett and Sawyer, 1950). Continuous treatment of ovariectomized rats with oestradiol elicited ovulatory-type spikes of plasma LH at the same time on successive afternoons (Legan and Karsch, 1975). Therefore, the neural signal is a daily event and requires oestrogen for expression at the pituitary level. The signal triggers the release of LHRH from nerve terminals in the median eminence of the hypothalamus to bring about the ovulatory surge of pituitary gonadotrophins (Sarkar *et al.*, 1976; Levine and Ramirez, 1982). However, the magnitude of the increase of LHRH in pituitary portal blood during the critical period is insufficient to explain the entire output of pituitary hormones, which must also depend upon rising sensitivity of gonadotrophs to LHRH (Aiyer *et al.*, 1974).

The timing of the critical period, which precedes ovulation by about 12 hr, is obviously an adaptation in this nocturnal species. The pacemaker is located in the rostral hypothalamus close to the suprachiasmatic nucleus, from which many circadian rhythms emanate. This location was demonstrated by the ability of bilateral lesions at the caudal margin of the optic chiasm to inhibit ovulatory surges of gonadotrophins. Basal hormone levels and follicular maturation remained unaffected by the lesions (Szentágothai et al., 1962; Blake et al., 1972). These results imply that gonadotrophin release in rats is under dual hypothalamic control. A rostral area is responsible for "cyclic" release whereas a medial basal area (the "hypophysiotrophic area") maintains "tonic" secretion in the absence of extrinsic neural inputs. The stimulatory or so-called positive feedback effects of oestradiol are exerted at the rostral site (Goodman, 1978) but require neuronal connections with the basal hypothalamus for releasing LH (Tejasen and Everett, 1967).

General concepts of hormonal feedback in the ovarian cycle apply equally in rodents and primates (Fig. 2.3), but the hierarchical organization of glandular control mechanisms are different. Despite continuing controversy, recent evidence provides strong indications that the rhesus monkey ovary provides its own timing mechanism for the events of the menstrual cycle, rather than depending on a circadian rhythm generator in the brain. Neither the blood levels of gonadotrophins nor the hourly frequency ("circhoral") with which they rise were affected by surgical disconnection of nerves projecting to the medial basal hypothalamus (Krey et al., 1975). In contrast to the aforementioned effects of these lesions in rats, the normal response of the primate pituitary gland to positive feedback effects of oestradiol was unaffected. These findings explain why the timing of the mid-cycle surge of gonadotrophins in primates is less obviously dependent on a circadian rhythm and why it is not interrupted by barbiturate anaesthesia. The emergent concept from these discoveries is that the ovary is the "clock" for the menstrual cycle, each phase being determined by the time taken to build an ovulatory follicle or destroy a corpus luteum (Knobil, 1974). This mechanism is in striking contrast to the cerebral clock of rats, which is coupled to the photoperiodic cycle (Everett, 1974).

Despite this progress towards understanding the physiology of the menstrual cycle, some difficulties remain. If the hypothalamus simply "drips" LHRH onto the underlying pituitary gland, then a role for the brain in processing interoceptive and exteroceptive inputs is abrogated. This apparent theoretical obstacle is diminished if the magnitude or frequency of LHRH pulses can be modulated (see later). Of even greater concern is the conflicting experimental finding of another highly respected research group. Norman et al. (1976), using a different technique for isolating the basal hypothalamus in monkeys, found that disruption of pathways from the preoptic area–anterior hypothalamus abolished ovulatory function and feedback control. However, Ferin et al. (1977) obtained evidence supporting the original findings, which have been extended by Knobil's group using a different approach. To identify the site of oestradiol feedback, the latter group abolished pituitary stimulation by endogenous LHRH by producing radio-frequency lesions in the hypothalamic arcuate nucleus. After treatment, it was necessary to infuse LHRH in pulses at hourly intervals in order to maintain physiological levels of gonadotrophins and pituitary responsiveness to oestrogen (Fig. 4.1). These pulses are thought to mimic the natural rhythm of neurosecre-

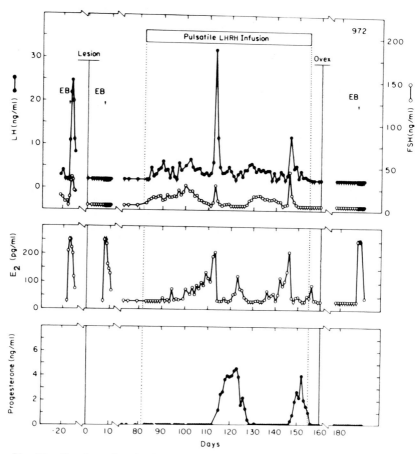

Fig. 4.1. Experimental study of the role of LHRH and gonadal steroids in the control of the menstrual cycle in rhesus monkeys. See text for details. EB, oestradiol benzoate; Ovex, bilateral ovariectomy; Lesion, hypothalamic lesion to disrupt secretion of endogenous LHRH. [Reprinted with permission from E. Knobil, T. M. Plant, L. Wildt, P. E. Belchetz and G. Marshall (1980), Control of the rhesus monkey menstrual cycle: Permissive role of hypothalamic gonadotropin-releasing hormone, *Science* **207**, 1371–1373; Copyright 1980 by the AAAS.]

tion which is responsible for oscillation of pituitary hormone release (Clarke and Cummins, 1982). This infusion maintained follicular maturation and ovulation, as witnessed by successive increases of endogenous oestradiol and progesterone. Two major discharges of gonadotrophins occurred at an interval of about 1 month. This decisively proves that normal cyclic activity and feedback relationships in monkeys do not require mediation by release of hypothalamic LHRH. It is therefore no longer surprising that oestradiol elicits a surge of gonadotrophins when endogenous LHRH is neutralized with antibodies (McCormack et al., 1977; Fraser et al., 1984). Oestradiol can exert its actions as much as 48 hr after eliminating LHRH; thus, it too must be a gonadotrophin-releasing hormone (Wildt et al., 1981a).

Details concerning the control of ovarian cycles are available for few species, yet it is clear already that talk of ''animal models'' is hazardous. Ovarian cycles in ageing rodents can (and do) cease for reasons which differ from those in primates because they are controlled by different physiological mechanisms. Knowledge of the human menstrual cycle is bound to depend heavily on animal research, and the rhesus monkey provides the best available model at present. Cycles in the two species are similar in terms of phase lengths and circulating hormone profiles, but some differences exist (e.g. absence of a luteal phase oestrogen peak in monkeys) (Knobil, 1974). Clinical studies have shown that infusion of LHRH or its analogues in pulses every 60–120 min is sufficient to restore ovulation in patients with hypogonadotrophic amenorrhoea (Yen, 1983). If hypothalamic function is ''permissive'' as far as the control of human ovulation is concerned, we gain a new perspective in our understanding of events leading towards the menopause.

4.3. Patterns of Cyclical Activity throughout Life

Laboratory Rodents

Rodents' short lifespan and low cost, as well as the ease of recording their cycles by the vaginal smear technique, make them ideal subjects for study of the effects of ageing. Several longitudinal studies of ovarian cycles in rodents have been published.

The most comprehensive study involved inbred mice of the C57BL/6J strain aged 3–18 months (Nelson et al., 1982). Three phases of the lifespan were delineated according to the regularity of oestrous activity: I: an initial phase of relatively infrequent and irregular cycles in which cycle frequency increased linearly with age; II: a phase of maximum cycle frequency and stability; III: a phase of steadily declining cycle frequency (Fig. 4.2). The transition time between these phases varied within the ranges 3.5–4.5 and 10.5–13.5 months in

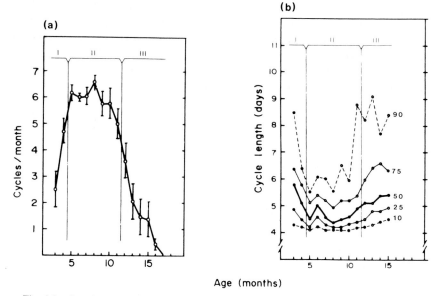

Fig. 4.2. Longitudinal study of oestrous cycles in virgin C57BL/6J mice (cohort A). (a) Average monthly cycle frequency. (b) Median and selected percentile values for cycle length. In each case three phases are shown: ascending (I), peak (II) and declining (III) periods of cycle frequency. (From Nelson *et al.*, 1982.)

different cohorts of animals. Cycle lengths were shortest during phase II, but they were not precise reciprocals of cycle frequency because the latter is a global measurement, including individuals that stop cycling as well as those with genuine changes of cycle length. The normal oestrous cycle of young rodents lasts only 4 or 5 days because corpora lutea are inactive unless mating has occurred. Surprisingly, there is less uniformity amongst mice than amongst rats and "strings" of short cycles of the same length are not particularly common, despite genetic uniformity in inbred mice. The frequency of consecutive pairs of 4- and 5-day cycles in C57BL/6J mice was maximal for a short time in phase II. The longer cycles of the other phases resulted from additional days of either vaginal cornification or leucocytosis, reflecting different underlying endocrine states.

Formerly, it was thought that oestrous cycles in rodents continue into extreme old age, but many strains have now been shown to become acyclical in mid-life, at 12–18 months. This difference is probably attributable to the combined effects of (1) the greater tendency today to use inbred strains in which reproductive life is shorter and (2) better husbandry conditions which prolong survival. The C57BL/6J strain has a long postreproductive phase of life. Animals become acyclical at 13–16 months of age, although ovulation is still a possibility and the ovaries continue to produce moderate amounts of oestrogen acyclically for several more months. In contrast, healthy males of the same strain maintain production of testosterone into extreme old age (Nelson *et al.*, 1975).

Oestrous cycles in rats follow patterns similar to those in mice. Cycle length is extended during ageing and days of vaginal cornification become more frequent, eventually replacing the normal cyclic pattern (Huang and Meites, 1975). In virgin rats of the now extinct inbred DA strain, persistent vaginal cornification ("persistent oestrus") began at only 4–5 months (Everett, 1939), but in most outbred animals it occurs at 6–12 months (Nelson *et al.*, 1982) and is slightly later in multiparous compared to virgin animals (Nass *et al.*, 1982). Persistent oestrus in rats frequently lasts for months and is followed by a phase of repetitive pseudopregnancy-like cycles and, finally, anoestrus (Bloch and Flury, 1959; Huang and Meites, 1975; Aschheim, 1976; Lu *et al.*, 1979). Spontaneous restoration of ovarian cycles, albeit infertile ones, following a prolonged anovulatory phase is not paralleled in women nor is it found in some strains of mice which are anoestrous for the greater part of postreproductive life (e.g. CBA, C57BL/6J).

Human and Other Primates

Cycle Length

The first carefully documented record of the frequency of human menses was published by Clos (1858). Like other workers in the nineteenth century, he was preoccupied with the supposed association with phases of the moon. His data are of interest today only because they portend the results of modern large-scale studies of the effects of ageing.

In 1967, Treloar *et al.* published a major longitudinal study of menstrual histories between adolescence and menopause. This monumental work involved Caucasian women enrolled at the University of Minnesota, who recorded personal details of vaginal bleeding, contraception, reproductive events and medical history continuously over many years. The project began in 1934 and progressively involved about 5000 women. Concurrently, Vollman (1977) was collating similar records of 691 Swiss women attending a general practice together with additional information about the frequency of ovulatory cycles estimated from nonspecific criteria, viz. rectal temperature, cervical mucorrhoea and intermenstrual pain. The results of these two independent studies are remarkably consistent.

When the average length of menstrual cycles was plotted against either chronological or gynaecological age (i.e. from menarche), J- or U-shaped curves were obtained (Fig. 4.3). The distribution of cycle lengths was skewed, and median values, which were lower than means, were more meaningful descriptions of

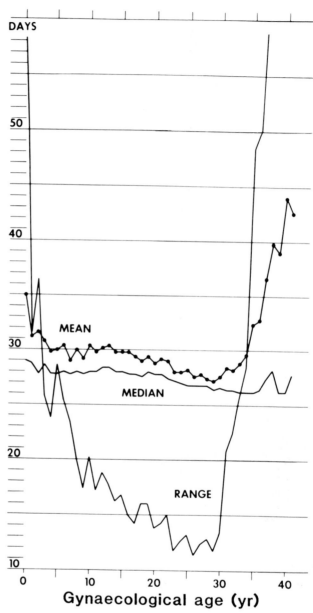

Fig. 4.3. Variation in the length of menstrual cycle from menarche (age 0) to menopause. A total of 30,261 cycles were reported by 594 women. (From Vollman, 1977; reprinted with permission.)

central tendency. In the American study, the distributions were divided into three zones (postmenarcheal, middle and premenopausal) for the entire menstrual span of 36 years (Treloar *et al.*, 1967). Throughout this span the celebrated 28-day cycle tends to be modal at most ages (Fig. 4.4). Variation of cycle length is more striking when plotted according to gynaecological rather than chronological age, perhaps because values begin at a uniform stage of biological maturation. Beginning at a median of 29 days at menarche, cycle length descends steadily to 26 days at age 40 in Swiss women (gynaecological ages quoted) (Fig. 4.3). Mean values fall steeply from 35 to 30 days between ages 0 and 4. Subsequent descent is more gradual until a nadir of 27 days is reached at 29 years, this decrease being due exclusively to shorter follicular phases. Finally, there is a steep ascent to 44 days at the close of menstrual life. The frequency distribution of cycles of specified length is both complex and continuous (Fig. 4.4). During the postmenarcheal zone, cycles >29 days long tend to decline in frequency, whilst shorter cycles are steady. The pattern changes at 7 years (about 21–22 years chronologically) when short cycles (<24 days) are replaced abruptly by 25- to 28-day cycles. Further changes are seen from 30 years (or about 45 chronologically), shorter cycles becoming more common and longer ones declining correspondingly. In the final years of menstrual life, cycles 21–35 days long become less frequent, whereas very short (<21 days) and very long cycles (>35 days) comprise nearly half of all cycles.

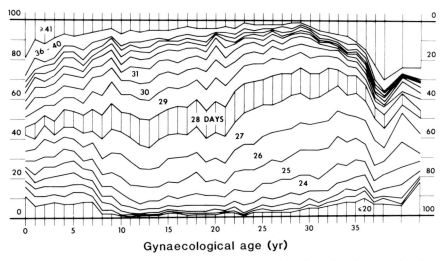

CUMULATIVE PERCENTAGES

Fig. 4.4. Cumulative percentage distribution of the individual lengths of menstrual cycles according to gynaecological age in women. (From Vollman, 1977; reprinted with permission.)

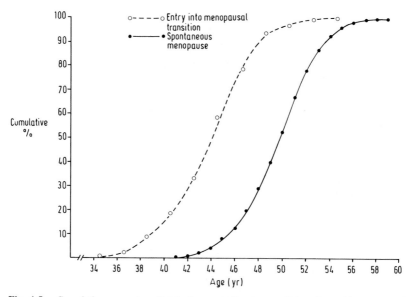

Fig. 4.5. Cumulative percentage distribution according to age of American white women who reached the menopausal transition (*n* = 291) and menopause (*n* = 393). (From Treloar, 1981; reprinted with permission.)

Thus, the range of cycle lengths is greatest near the beginning and end of menstrual life (Fig. 4.3); minimal variation is seen at a chronological age of 36 years (Treloar *et al.*, 1967). The zone of irregular cycles preceding the menopause has been called the "menopausal transition." It lasts about 6–8 years and its length is mostly independent of age at onset, although it is slightly shorter in women attaining a late menopause (Fig. 4.5). It is these women who have the greatest variation and extension of cycle length in the final two years of menses, and these factors might be responsible for their higher risk of breast cancer (Wallace *et al.*, 1978).

Similar changes in menstrual cyclicity might be expected in sub-human primates, but data are rare. In a longitudinal study, van Wagenen (1972) observed three rhesus monkeys with oligomenorrhoea in their third decade of life. At ages 27 and 28 years, two of them finally stopped cycling, having evidently reached menopause (Fig. 4.6).

In conclusion, longitudinal studies show that menstrual life is not simply switched on at menarche and off at menopause with an intervening phase of regular cycles. As in rodents, there are continuous changes in frequency of ovarian cycles, signifying underlying changes of maturation and senescence of the reproductive system. It is anticipated that parallel changes will be found for other parameters, as indicated in the next section.

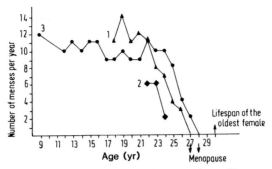

Fig. 4.6. Climacteric and menopause in three rhesus monkeys. (From van Wagenen, 1972; reprinted with permission.)

Cycle Quality

The quality of menstrual cycles is generally studied by measuring basal body temperature and steroid excretion rates since more direct and precise methods involving plasma hormone assay are difficult to organize in large-scale surveys and repeated venepuncture is stressful.

The incidence of abnormal cycles is shown in Table 4.1. Cycles with a hyperthermic phase of <10 days were considered infertile, and those lacking an obvious mid-cycle rise in temperature were presumed to be anovulatory (Döring, 1963). Such cycles occur at all ages, but they are most frequent near the beginning and ending of the menstrual lifespan (Collett *et al.*, 1954; Vollman, 1977; Metcalf and MacKenzie, 1980).

Longitudinal studies of urinary hormone profiles in perimenopausal women in New Zealand provide a rare glimpse at the underlying patterns of ovarian changes. Women aged 36–55 years were selected soon after a break in their natural menstrual rhythms, and they collected weekly specimens of urine for steroid and gonadotrophin analysis (Metcalf *et al.*, 1981a). Two main types of cycle were identified: (1) "short" cycles <45 days in length, in which gonadotrophin excretion was normal with a pronounced rise of pregnanediol, indicating ovulation; these cycles occurred sporadically up to 16 weeks before the last menses (Metcalf *et al.*, 1981b); (2) highly abnormal cycles in which gonadotrophin excretion rates rose to the postmenopausal range for long periods of up to 8 months, sometimes associated with hot flushes. Thus, the probability of ovulation in any cycle is related more closely to cycle length than to age (Metcalf, 1979, 1983).

Elongated cycles are experienced by most perimenopausal women. They tend to be anovular with highly variable patterns of hormone excretion, but FSH and oestrogen are frequently elevated simultaneously for several weeks (van Look *et al.*, 1977; Metcalf and Donald, 1979). Thus, the menopause is heralded by a

TABLE 4.1

The Proportion of Abnormal Menstrual Cycles during the Late Phase of the Reproductive Lifespan in Women

	Source: Döring (1963)				Source: Vollman (1977)		
Age (years)	Anovulatory cycles (%)	Cycles with short luteal phase (%)[a]	Total abnormal cycles (%)	Approx. age[b] (years)	Anovulatory cycles (%)	Cycles with short luteal phase (%)[a]	Total abnormal cycles (%)
31–35	7	9	16	30–34	3	10	13
36–40	3	16	19	35–39	2	9	11
41–45	12	18	30	40–44	4	12	16
46–50	15	36	51	≥45	18	12	30

[a] <10 days.

[b] The original data set has been retabulated and is approximate because it was tabulated according to gynaecological age rather than chronological age (after Gray, 1979).

high output of gonadotrophins in advance of the profound and sustained fall in ovarian secretion (Metcalf *et al.*, 1982). The causes of prolonged secretion of oestrogen are not understood, though it seems likely that altered feedback relationships are at fault, with implications for follicular dynamics. Either dominant follicle(s) fail to become atretic after a normal period of preovulatory secretion or an unbroken succession of these types form. As a consequence of persistent secretion of oestrogen without opposing effects of progesterone, there is an increased probability of dysfunctional uterine bleeding among women of perimenopausal age (de Jong *et al.*, 1974).

When urinary assays are used, subtle changes of endocrine function are likely to go unnoticed. Even before cycles become irregular, blood hormone measurements can indicate that the climacteric is imminent in women of middle age (Fig. 4.7). The hormone profiles are generally similar to those of younger women, but peak levels of oestradiol are lower during the follicular and luteal phases, whilst FSH levels are increased at most times of the cycle (Sherman *et al.*, 1976; van Look *et al.*, 1977). In rhesus monkeys, similar changes occur during the climacteric (Hodgen *et al.*, 1977; Dierschke *et al.*, 1983). Reyes *et al.* (1977) found circulating levels of LH and progesterone during the menstrual cycle tended to fall during ageing, but these findings have not been confirmed in other studies. Since pituitary production of FSH and LH depends on stimulation by the same neuropeptide, LHRH, it is conjectured that differential elevation of FSH is caused by lower output of follicular inhibin by ageing ovaries. This counterpart of testicular inhibin is capable of suppressing secretion of FSH (de Jong and Sharpe, 1976), but its physiological significance requires clarification.

The peculiar features of perimenopausal cycles are too variable to provide a practical basis for predicting the final menses. Urinary gonadotrophic activity may be elevated for weeks and is indistinguishable from that of the postmenopause. Oestrogenic activity is not a better guide since it fluctuates during the first few months after the menopause as a few remaining follicles make fruitless attempts to mature. The endocrine data confirm that the changes of the menopausal transition are not abrupt but rather involve the progressive loss of ovarian function.

The University of Minnesota study of menstrual histories has provided a limited basis for predicting the timing of menopause for the North American white population (Fig. 4.8). Variation in the probability that menopause has occurred has been plotted against the first record of amenorrhoea of given duration. The relationship is approximately linear, but the probability of menopause is higher at each point on the abscissa for older women. For example, there is a 13% chance that menopause has occurred at the first interval of 90–119 days of amenorrhoea in 47-year-old women, but the corresponding value is 30% at age 51 and 47% at age 54. Even after a year without menses, there is a residual 5–10% chance that vaginal bleeding will occur, assuming this is not due to genital

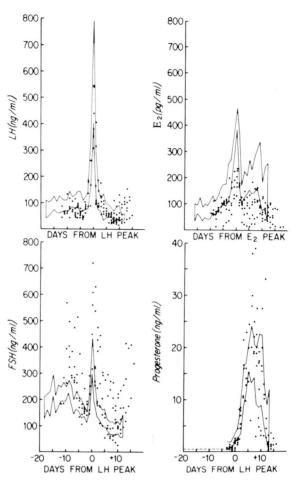

Fig. 4.7. Serum concentrations of LH, FSH, oestradiol (E_2) and progesterone during menstrual cycles of women aged 46–56 years compared with values (mean $\pm$ 2 SEM) of women aged 18–30 (enclosed area). Data have been normalized for the day of the LH peak. (From Sherman *et al.*, 1976; reprinted with permission.)

tract disease or withdrawal of exogenous hormones. This illustrates the probabilistic nature of conventional criteria of menopause.

4.4. Aetiology of Acyclicity and Menopause

A great deal is known about the biology of ageing in rodents. Strictly speaking, these animals cannot have a menopause, but they do have patterns of

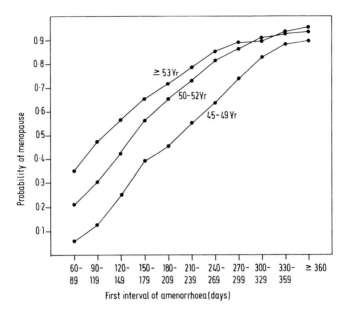

Fig. 4.8. Variation in probability of menopause according to the length of amenorrhoea in American whites. Three curves have been plotted to show the effects of age. [From R. B. Wallace, B. M. Sherman, J. A. Bean, A. E. Treloar and L. Schlabaugh (1979), Probability of menopause with increasing duration of amenorrhea in middle-aged women, *Am. J. Obstet. Gynecol.* **135,** 1021–1024.]

reproductive senescence that are common to many species, including our own. Therefore, it is appropriate to begin by discussing the causes of ovarian ageing in rodents and then to compare and contrast the human menopause.

Balance of Factors in Rodents: Ovarian or Neuroendocrine?

Waning reproductive function in animals was formerly attributed to "wearing out" of ovaries. This view seemed to be upheld by the discovery that the follicular store is non-renewable, but it was rejected when significant numbers of follicles were found in postreproductive mice (Jones, 1970). There is now abundant evidence that extra-ovarian factors are at least partly responsible for failure of ovulation in ageing rodents.

The relative responsibilities of central versus peripheral factors in ovarian senescence have been weighed by means of ovarian transplantation experiments. If ovarian ageing limits the length of cyclical life, then replacement by younger ovaries should restore function. However, the first reports in rats showed that senile animals did not return to normal oestrous cycles after organ replacement, whereas old ovaries were revitalized in young hosts, showing that responsive follicles remained (Aschheim, 1964–1965; Peng and Huang, 1972). Consequently, it was concluded that the ageing hypothalamo-pituitary unit is incapable of releasing ovulatory amounts of gonadotrophins even though its secretory activity is adequate for follicular growth and maturation.

When similar transplantation experiments were carried out with C57BL/6J mice, the balance of responsibility was found to be more complex (Felicio *et al.*, 1983). Ovaries from young donor mice aged 5 months were grafted under renal capsules of ovariectomized hosts aged 5–30 months. The profiles of ovarian cycles which followed in the young–young combination and intact controls were similar, the only notable difference being earlier termination of cycles in the grafted animals, and this could be accounted for by ischaemic necrosis of follicles whilst grafts became established (Fig. 4.9). When ovaries were grafted into hosts of postcyclic age (17 months), cycles were restored for a shorter period of 3 months at 25% of control levels. Grafts showed even less cyclical activity in older hosts. These results indicate that ovulatory function is limited by ageing of the neuroendocrine control mechanisms in the host. Concurrent studies tested whether the feeble activity of young grafts in ageing mice was affected by the earlier history of endocrine function in the hosts. Tentative evidence of improved graft performance in long-term ovariectomized rats had been presented already (Aschheim, 1964–1965). This was confirmed in mice by finding that the number of cycles produced by grafts in hosts deprived of their own ovaries between 5 and 17 months approached that of 5-month-old controls. There were, however, fewer cycles amongst older hosts (Fig. 4.9).

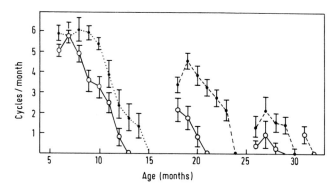

Fig. 4.9. Experimental study of effects of the age of the host and the duration of ovariectomy on the ability of ovarian grafts to restore oestrous cycles in ageing C57BL/6J mice. Grafts were obtained from young donor animals aged 3–5 months and inserted under renal capsules of syngeneic hosts at one of the following ages: 5, 17, 25, 30 months. The hosts had been ovariectomized either shortly before receiving grafts (O- - -O) or after a prolonged period of ovariectomy beginning at 5 months of age (•- - -•). An additional group of mice with their ovaries intact served as control (•···•). Means ± SEM are shown. (From Felicio *et al.*, 1983.)

In conclusion, at least three groups of factors limit cyclical activity in these ageing mice. (1) Primary ovarian ageing is indicated by the ability of grafts to restore oestrous cycles. Similar conclusions were reached by Krohn (1962) in pioneering experiments with CBA mice, in which ovarian failure occurs in mid-life. (2) Extra-ovarian factors must be operating because graft activity was improved in long-term ovariectomized hosts. They might involve actions of ovarian hormones on hypothalamo-pituitary function. (3) Other extra-ovarian factors that are independent of the history of ovarian activity finally limit the maximum cycle extension in the lifespan. Since this limit is reached late in life, general debilitation might be responsible.

We can see then that a number of factors are operating in mice to bring about acyclicity, whereas in rats the hypothalamus (and possibly the pituitary gland) has been held to be wholly responsible. Nevertheless, there is now evidence that in Holtzman rats ovarian ageing is a contributing factor (Sopelak and Butcher, 1982), which shows we cannot simply assign species-specific causes of acyclicity. Future research should aim to elucidate how genetic and environmental variables influence the balance of factors which bring about the onset of reproductive senescence.

Hormone Production and Feedback in Ageing Rodents

Age-related changes in reproductive hormone levels begin in mice at 10–13 months of age when cycles are lengthening (Fig. 4.10). Peak preovulatory levels of oestradiol are undiminished though they begin their ascent later, perhaps because fewer follicles are recruited. The characteristic rise of progesterone on the periovulatory days is smaller, as is the ovulatory discharge of LH in both mice and rats (Cooper et al., 1980; Flurkey et al., 1982; Wise, 1982a). Most studies indicate that FSH secretion is not affected by ageing until after the time when ovarian cycles are disrupted. Progressive impedance of the mechanism for releasing LH is not a significant factor at younger ages because blood hormone levels rise far higher than are required for ovulation and the number of ova shed per cycle is not diminished until acyclicity is imminent. Nevertheless, this change is a notable indication of neuroendocrine dysfunction leading to anovulation with persistent oestrus in mid-life.

The ovaries of anovulatory rats and mice presenting persistent vaginal cornification are dominated by large Graafian follicles (Fig. 3.13). Since corpora lutea are absent, blood levels of progesterone and 20α-dihydroprogesterone are low. Apart from minor diurnal fluctuations, there are no cyclical rhythms of reproductive hormone levels. Plasma oestradiol levels are intermediate between those of castrates and cyclic animals at pro-oestrus (Lu et al., 1979; Felicio et al., 1980). The gonadotrophins are not substantially elevated. Steady and prolonged output of oestrogen, unopposed by progesterone, has pathological significance (Fig.

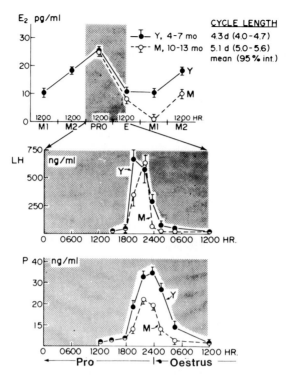

Fig. 4.10. Changes in plasma hormone levels during oestrous cycles in young (Y) and middle-aged (M) C57BL/6J mice. Top panel: oestradiol (E₂) was similar in Y and M at pro-oestrus, but fell to lower values in M. Middle panel: LH rose more slowly to peak values and subsequently declined more rapidly in M; basal levels were similar in both groups. Bottom panel: peak levels of progesterone (P) were lower in M than Y. (From Finch *et al.*, 1980; reprinted with permission.)

4.11). Frequently, it leads to cystic glandular hyperplasia with fibrosis in the uterus. Furthermore, it stimulates mammotrophs which hypertrophy and produce prolactin copiously. Hyperprolactinaemia leads to galactorrhoea and tumours in mammary glands of susceptible animal strains. Unless exhaustion of the follicular store intervenes, increasing output of prolactin will lead eventually to luteinization of mature follicles and, hence, pseudopregnancy cycles later in life. Gonadal secretion will then change to a pattern of lower levels of oestrogens combined with high, fluctuating amounts of progestogens (Lu *et al.*, 1979). The final, irreversible state of vaginal anoestrus in some mouse strains resembles the postmenopausal phase of women in some respects. Vaginal anoestrus signifies a deficiency of ovarian follicles and oestrogen. In the absence of feedback restraint, the gonadotrophs hypertrophy and plasma levels of gonadotrophins increase (Parkening *et al.*, 1980; Gee *et al.*, 1983). The lack of comparable changes in rats might be attributable to elevated prolactin in this species.

Loss of ovarian cycles in mid-life is associated with reduced central responsiveness to gonadal steroids, as shown by the inability of native or grafted ovaries to elicit ovulatory amounts of gonadotrophins. Defective positive feedback has also been demonstrated using ovariectomized animals by mimicking the endogenous hormonal changes with exogenous steroids. The amount of LH released by exogenous oestrogen or progesterone in rats primed with oestrogen has been shown repeatedly to be diminished in middle-aged compared with younger rats (see Blake *et al.*, 1983). Impaired positive feedback responses to gonadal steroids are not restricted to this species but have been recorded in other rodents and even in the domestic fowl (Williams and Sharp, 1978). Whereas failure of positive feedback might be a general feature of ageing, there is little convincing evidence of impaired negative feedback responses to these steroids. It is widely presumed, though not yet proven by direct measurement, that inability to release sufficient LHRH is responsible for attenuated feedback effects.

Since physical and chemical lesions of the rostral hypothalamus lead to positive feedback failure and anovulation (Blake *et al.*, 1972; Benedetti *et al.*, 1976), this site is held to be responsible for the spontaneous loss of oestrous cycles. In support of this hypothesis, electrical stimulation of the preoptic area (or arcuate nucleus) stimulates ovulation in acyclic rats, though fewer ova are shed than in normal cycles. The amounts of LH released in these experiments indicated that pools of readily releasible LHRH and LH are adequate and that gonadotrophs are sufficiently sensitive (Everett and Tyrey, 1983). However, the question of pituitary responsiveness to LHRH is still unsettled, and further study is required to clarify conflicting claims. Where reduced responsiveness has been observed, it is attributed to the effects of ovarian secretions rather than to chronological ageing *per se* (Cooper *et al.*, 1984).

Our limited knowledge of the basic physiology of hypothalamic function holds back progress in understanding age changes. It is attractive to consider whether loss of hypothalamic sensitivity to feedback information is due to a reduced concentration of nuclear receptors for oestradiol, which has been observed in the preoptic area (Wise and Camp, 1984), other age changes in the neuroendocrine apparatus being secondary effects of this. Target neurons for feedback of oestradiol are probably not the same as those which synthesize and transport LHRH from the rostral hypothalamus to the site of release in the median eminence (Shivers *et al.*, 1983). Monoaminergic synapses are involved at unidentified stages in the neural pathways for both circadian and pulsatile release of gonadotrophins. Because of their position in the hierarchical organization, small changes in the activity of hypothalamic monoamines could create a cascade of functional disturbances at lower levels and in peripheral organs (Finch, 1976). This potential is illustrated by the serious effects on motor control of altered dopaminergic functions in ageing basal ganglia (Finch *et al.*, 1981) and by the restoration of ovarian cycles by centrally acting drugs (see below). Hence, it may be significant that both concentrations and metabolism of noradrenaline are reduced in anterior hypothalami of ageing female rats (Meites *et al.*, 1982; Wise, 1982b). Levels of other putative neurotransmitter and neuromodulator substances may vary in middle age, but this catecholamine is of particular interest because of its probable involvement in releasing LHRH (Simpkins *et al.*, 1979; Gallo and Kalra, 1983).

The hypothesis that altered neuronal activity contributes to the acyclicity of ageing is strengthened by the discovery that exogenous agents restore function. Progesterone was the first substance shown to have this effect, which was obtained after administration in small, repeated doses (Everett, 1940). To conclude from this that anovulatory rats must therefore have a deficiency of this hormone is too superficial since it avoids the question of how luteinization failed in the first place. Progesterone probably restores cycles by alleviating the insensitivity of the brain to oestrogen. Alternative explanations may have to be found for the efficacy of other agents, such as noradrenaline, dopaminergic agonists, ether stress, ACTH (Quadri *et al.*, 1973; Huang *et al.*, 1976), dietary supplements of L-tyrosine (Linnoila and Cooper, 1976) and decreasing photoperiod (Everett, 1970). The ability of catecholamine precursors to restore cycles when administered directly to the preoptic area supports the general belief that neuronal function in this area becomes defective in old animals (Cooper and Linnoila, 1980).

Although these experiments provide *prima facie* evidence of altered neuroendocrine function, it is important to appreciate the possibilities of cycle restoration by non-specific means. Restoration by substances given on a daily basis might be explained by the reinforcement of a circadian rhythm which has become damped during ageing (e.g. the adrenal rhythm) (Mosko *et al.*, 1980). Treatments which produce only a single cycle should not be assumed to have affected the causes of acyclicity, and there may be more than one possible interpretation of cycle restoration. When a set of corpora lutea are introduced by any stimulus, momentum may be created for a series of short cycles in which luteal progesterone facilitates cyclic release of LH. The response to treatment then depends on endogenous levels of prolactin (which is luteotrophic) rather than continuation of exogenous agents. If prolactin levels are low, the anovulatory state is quickly resumed; if they are higher, a longer series of cycles commences. In rats with pituitary tumours secreting prolactin abundantly, short cycles may switch to the longer pseudopregnancy type (Everett, 1980).

The timing of loss of sensitivity to positive feedback depends upon the earlier history of ovarian secretions. This is evident from the ovarian transplantation experiments cited earlier and has been confirmed by the improved pituitary response to gonadal steroids in animals deprived of ovaries over a long period (Lu *et al.*, 1981; Blake *et al.*, 1983). Since long-term ovariectomy protects hypothalamo-pituitary function from deleterious effects of ageing, can excessive exposure to oestradiol early in adulthood accelerate the loss of cycles? An affirmative answer was obtained when intact adult rats were treated with large doses of oestradiol valerate (Brawer *et al.*, 1978). Their arcuate nuclei had histopathological changes indicative of neuronal damage (viz. hyperactive glia). Similar changes occurred spontaneously during ageing (Brawer *et al.*, 1980) and could be induced by physiological levels of oestrogen (Mobbs *et al.*, 1984). In either case, loss of ovarian cycles could not be explained by pituitary tumours but may have been due to defective function of LHRH-containing neurons.

A heuristic model has been proposed to explain the loss of cycles during

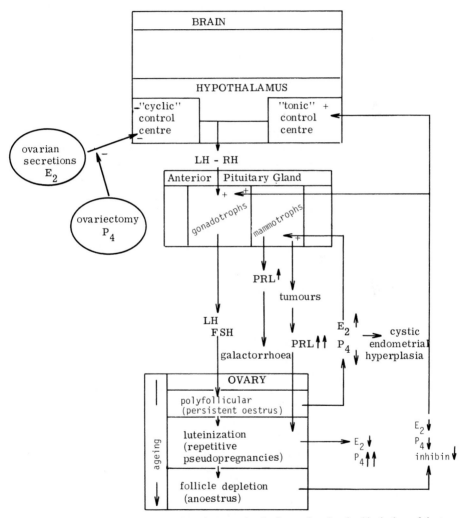

Fig. 4.11. Schematic representation of neuroendocrine interactions involved in the loss of short ovulatory cycles in ageing rodents. Some pathological consequences of anovulation are shown: +, stimulation or lack of inhibition; −, inhibition; ↑, increased production; ↓, decreased production; E_2, oestradiol; P_4, progesterone.

ageing and after oestrogen treatment (Finch *et al.,* 1980). Exposure of the rodent brain to gonadal steroids (particularly oestrogen) throughout life may lead to accumulated damage, and at some critical threshold, the mechanism of cyclic release of LH is impaired because of insensitivity to oestradiol. The threshold would be attained later in animals lacking ovaries or exposed to progesterone over a long period. Although a neural "memory" of oestrogen stimulation is hypothetical for the present, the model which is emerging is consistent with the general picture of reproductive system ageing in which complex interactions exist at different levels, making hazardous any attempts to assign strict hierarchical responsibility for dysfunction (Fig. 4.11).

Human Menopause

Human menopause is usually presented as a comparatively more straightforward case of peripheral organ failure. There is little doubt that primary ovarian ageing brings about the final cessation of menses, although closer study of the physiology suggests that other complex changes occur during the perimenopause. Few follicles remain in the postmenopausal ovary, and they fail to mature despite abundant circulating gonadotrophins of proven biological activity (see Section 3.8). This circumstance prohibits the restoration of cycles. The ability of monoamine precursors to reinitiate ovarian cycles in rats finds no convincing parallel in human biology, and reports of postmenopausal vaginal bleeding in women receiving levodopa (L-Dopa) should be explained on other grounds (Kruse-Larsen and Garde, 1971; Wajsbort, 1972). Conclusive proof that menstrual life is terminated by ovarian ageing could be obtained if normal cycles were resumed in postmenopausal women after grafting ovaries from young donors. However, such experiments are highly questionable from an ethical standpoint.

There are other grounds for supporting the "exhausted ovary" theory of human menopause and in particular the elevation of plasma gonadotrophins (Goldenberg *et al.,* 1973). Circulating levels of FSH and LH rise after menopause approximately 13- and 3-fold, respectively, compared with those of the early follicular phase in cyclic women (Figs. 4.12 and 4.13). Thus, levels of both gonadotrophins reach the castrate range, with FSH being the more abundant of the two. These high levels are maintained for at least 1 decade after menopause, though most studies have found that they fall in the last years of life (Wide *et al.,* 1973; Chakravarti *et al.,* 1976; Crilly *et al.,* 1981). In contrast to gonadotrophins, prolactin levels tend to fall slightly after menopause (Vekemans and Robyn, 1975). This is expected since the stimulatory effects of gonadal steroids on prolactin secretion are withdrawn at this time.

Increased blood levels of gonadotrophins are usually interpreted as a sign that the pituitary gland is no longer able to elicit a feedback response from atrophic ovaries. These elevated gonadotrophin levels are presumed to be due to rising

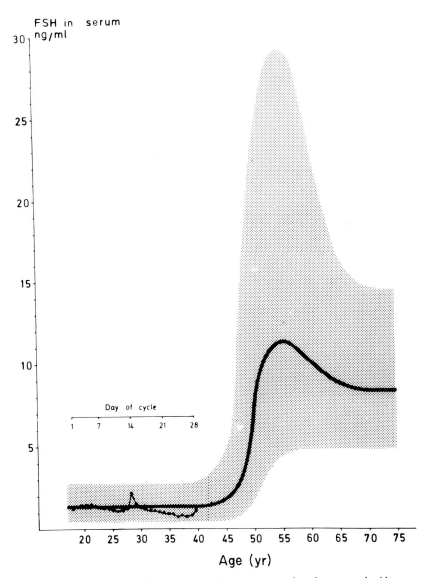

Fig. 4.12. Serum levels of FSH during the human menstrual cycle compared with average trends during ageing. (From Wide *et al.*, 1973; reprinted with permission.)

LH in serum
ng/ml

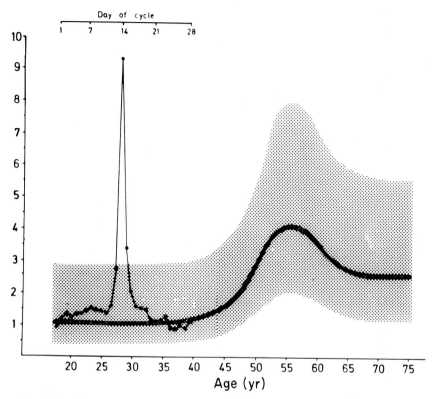

Fig. 4.13. Serum levels of LH during the human menstrual cycle compared with average trends during ageing. (From Wide *et al.*, 1973; reprinted with permission.)

concentrations of LHRH in pituitary portal blood, although dilution and rapid metabolism of LHRH during circulation have hampered attempts to obtain direct proof of this hypothesis. Hypothalamic levels of LHRH fall after menopause, but it is not possible to conclude whether this is due to more secretion or less synthesis of the decapeptide (Parker and Porter, 1984). Recent discoveries demand revision of classical concepts of feedback control and could significantly alter our view of postmenopausal gonadotrophins. It has been assumed that, since metabolic clearance rates do not change after menopause, increased blood levels of gonadotrophins reflect increased production (Kohler *et al.*, 1968; Coble *et al.*, 1969). This assumption must now be questioned because human and animal gonadotrophins have been shown to be pleiomorphic. Earlier measurements of hormone clearance rates in pre- and postmenopausal women employed the same standard hormone preparations, but such comparisons are misleading because different types of gonadotrophins circulate in these two groups. The types found in young women are less acidic than those in castrates, postmenopausal women and men (Wide, 1981, 1982; Reader et al., 1983). A smaller content of sialic acid is physiologically significant because it leads to more rapid clearance from blood, which would aid the fine control of follicular maturation by allowing prompt responses to feedback information (Wide and Hobson, 1983; Wide and Wide, 1984). The increasing acidity of FSH after the menopause seems to be due to withdrawal of sex steroids, but such changes would appear to develop sluggishly, and they do not account for variable hormone levels during the normal menstrual cycle (Wide, 1982). Such findings do not call into question the present practice of using blood or urinary FSH activity as an indication of primary ovarian failure (Goldenberg et al., 1973). But it remains unclear whether the bulk of this activity is accounted for by increased production or decreased clearance of gonadotrophins.

The new concepts of how normal menstrual cycles are regulated endorse the current theory of the aetiology of menopause. In contrast to the situation in rodents, the human hypothalamus is unlikely to be responsible for acyclicity since it does not provide a stimulus for timing events in normal cycles. After menopause, pituitary responsiveness to LHRH remains and positive feedback responses to exogenous gonadal steroids are still possible (Odell and Swerdloff, 1968). Prolonged cycles during perimenopause are usually attributed to irregular recruitment from a dwindling pool of follicles, but primary ovarian ageing is not likely to account for shortening of the follicular phase during the middle zone of menstrual life. If this shortening is due to a greater growth velocity of the dominant follicle, it could be explained by frequency and/or amplitude modulation of LHRH pulses, perhaps rising abruptly before menarche (Wildt et al., 1980) and then more gradually during adult life. This explanation is purely hypothetical at the present time and will be difficult to test because pulses of FSH and, to a lesser extent, LH are difficult to quantify in women (Bäckström et al., 1982). But to continue this speculation, changes in neuronal activity in the hypothalamus could depend, in turn, on long-term changes in sensitivity to ovarian feedback, which have been postulated on other grounds (Dilman, 1971). In perimenopausal women, failure of oestrogen to exert positive feedback on LH release leads to anovulation with dysfunctional uterine bleeding (van Look et al., 1977, 1978). Experiments with rhesus monkeys show how this situation could arise as a result of decreased hypothalamic signal frequency. Following destruction of the pathway for endogenous release of LHRH, infusion of this peptide led to a rising FSH:LH ratio with irregular follicular maturation and anovulatory cycles when pulses were delivered at greater than the optimal interval of 1 hr (Wildt et al., 1981b; Pohl et al., 1983). These observations lead us to conjecture that there might be, after all, a link between perimenopausal changes in women and the neurohormonal basis of anovulation in rodents.

5

Fertility in Middle Age

5.1. Introduction

Twenty years ago, Krohn (1964) concluded from a far-reaching review of the literature that "there is no reasonable doubt, therefore, that (a) the likelihood of conceiving and (b) the size of a litter declines with increasing age in all the species for which there is any information at all". Subsequent studies have upheld his conclusion, although the number of species studied remains small and mainly confined to laboratory and domesticated groups.

A number of difficulties are encountered when measuring the effects of ageing on fertility and when designing gerontological experiments. The fertility of individuals of the same age and stock has a much larger coefficient of variation than most other physiological parameters (e.g. blood pressure, nerve conduction velocity), perhaps because individual survival does not depend on integrity of the reproductive apparatus. Furthermore, it is not always obvious whether infertility is due to normal and universal age changes ("eugeric" phenomena) rather than "pathogeric" changes which are secondary. For practical purposes, reproductive life in women is considered to begin at menarche and end at menopause, a span of 36 years in the developed world (Treloar, 1974). In contrast to wild animals, in which reproductive potential (fecundity) and actual performance (fertility) are closely matched, human fertility is modified by a host of factors which obscure any underyling trends of ageing. Some of the most significant of these are contraception, frequency of coitus, sterility of the male partner, age at marriage, prevalence of genital and other diseases, breast-feeding patterns and iatrogenic factors. It is the purpose of this chapter to review evidence for the age factor in human and animal reproduction, to discuss possible mechanisms and, finally, to reach some general conclusions of practical relevance for family planning in middle age.

5.2. Age-Specific Fertility

Animal Fertility

Small Laboratory Mammals

There have been many longitudinal studies of the fertility of laboratory mice, rats, hamsters and rabbits. Since these animals are polytocous (i.e. litter bearing), fluctuations in litter size throughout life provide an index of fertility. Control data in Fig. 5.9 show the number of offspring produced per uterine horn in outbred mice which were breeding *ad libitum* (total litter sizes are exactly double the values given). The age of sires was controlled because, although this variable does not affect litter size in mice (Finn, 1964), it may reduce the disposition to mate. The first litter is generally smaller than the second and, in some strains and species, peak litter size is not reached until the third or fourth pregnancy. This rise is mainly accounted for by increasing numbers of ovulations (p. 48). The phase of rising reproductive performance is followed by one of declining litter sizes which, towards the close of fertile life, is also characterized by less frequent deliveries (Asdell *et al.*, 1941; Ingram *et al.*, 1958; Jones and Krohn, 1961a; Soderwall *et al.*, 1960). Some researchers have shown an intermediate phase of relatively constant litter sizes in mice, but such findings depend on how the data are expressed. Fertility data often fit a three-phase model when a "standardized curve" is constructed (Biggers *et al.*, 1962). This manoeuvre was introduced to overcome statistical aberrations created by variation in the time when animals become infertile, but it rests on the assumption that fertility is lost for similar reasons in all individuals.

The length of fertile life is highly variable even among animals of a common stock. Reproduction commences at about 2–4 months of age in all the species named above and ceases 12 months later in most small rodents. Fertility is generally reduced by inbreeding in mice, but it rises in F_1 hybrids (Jones and Krohn, 1961a; Roberts, 1961). Since mice live for 2–3 years, they spend the second half of the lifespan in a postreproductive phase, which also exists in rats, hamsters, rabbits, gerbils and guinea pigs (Talbert, 1977).

Domesticated Animals

Despite their abundance, farm animals have provided scant data on fertility in old age because it is unprofitable to keep infertile stocks, and records which have been obtained are often biassed by selection for exceptional breeding performance. The available literature has been reviewed in depth by Krohn (1964) and Talbert (1977), who cautiously concluded that fertility decreases in ageing horses, cows, sheep and swine, as well as in cats and dogs. In view of artefacts that have been introduced by selective breeding practice in the past and in view of modern husbandry methods, it is not justifiable to extrapolate such conclusions to ancestral stocks of the same species or to extant wild relatives of domesticated animals. Reproductive senescence is rarely observed among wild animals because few survive long enough to become senescent. Even in species noted for longevity, such as African elephants, postreproductive individuals do not exist in wild populations (Perry, 1953).

Primates

Long-term fertility data for monkeys are scarce, but there are good prospects of future progress because the first animals to be born in U.S. primate research centres are now approaching the end of life. Information about great apes is presently limited to 10 chimpanzees aged 35–48 years, apart from isolated records from zoos and private collections. Although this group continued to have regular menstrual cycles until shortly before the end of life (about 50 years old), only three conceptions occurred and only one of these led to a live infant (Graham, 1979). The percentage of fertile menstrual cycles was only 4%, whereas it was 25% when the same animals were 15–25 years old. Longitudinal studies of breeding performance of lower primates are almost as rare as those of apes. In one colony, three rhesus monkeys reached menopause at ages 25–28, each having carried 12–14 pregnancies (van Wagenen, 1972). The oldest mother to deliver a live baby was 19 years old but required caesarian section, and there was a higher frequency of abortions and stillbirths among all older, multiparous mothers. However, these data may not be representative of the whole colony and could have been affected by earlier surgical procedures. This reservation is endorsed by a preliminary report from the Wisconsin Regional Primate Center that normal pregnancy in this species can occur as late as 26 years of age (Dierschke *et al.*, 1983).

Human Fertility

Live birth rates in Scotland are used to illustrate present fertility patterns in Western nations (Table 5.1). Fertility is much higher among women aged 25–29 years than in younger and older age groups. In the past, the age distribution for live births was bell-shaped (as it is today in many parts of the developing world); now it is skewed towards younger age groups. Apart from the greater frequency

TABLE 5.1

Age-Specific Fertility Rates of the Scottish Population, 1950 and 1980[a]

Age of mother (years)	Annual number of live births per 1000 women	
	1950	1980
15–19	20.98	32.52
20–24	128.59	112.65
25–29	147.77	130.54
30–34	108.16	67.30
35–39	60.88	20.49
40–44	18.16	3.73
45–49	1.26	0.18
15–49	69.86	63.82

[a] From the General Register Office, Scotland.

of teenage maternity, the fertility of all other age groups has fallen during the past 3 decades. The decline has been most rapid amongst older women. In 1950, women aged 40–49 were responsible for 4% of recorded deliveries in Scotland, whereas in 1980 they contributed only 1% of births. In many other countries similar patterns have been found, and though social and economic forces may bring about minor fluctuations, demographic forecasters expect these patterns will be maintained for at least the next 2 decades.Since demographic statistics from modern industrial societies cannot provide reliable estimates of human fecundity, it is necessary to turn to records from historical and traditional societies in which "natural fertility" has been less suppressed. Unfortunately, it is often these societies in which documentation of reproductive events and parental age is least satisfactory. Nevertheless, from a careful study of historical sources, Henry (1961) was able to conclude that fertility of married couples declined steadily from the third decade of life, approaching zero at age 50. This decline has been attributed to biological factors since it is remarkably similar in most societies that have been studied. Surveys of contemporary societies have shown that the average age at which fertility is lost (age at last live delivery) is about 40 (Gray, 1979), though it is earlier in places where gonorrhoea and genital tuber- culosis are widespread and in some undernourished societies (Scragg, 1973; Chavez and Martinez, 1982). Therefore, the average age of sterility precedes that of menopause by up to 10 years. The demographic data do not distinguish women who are sterile from those in whom residual fertile capacity exists; consequently, the exponential decrease in the proportion of sterile women by age (Pittenger, 1973) does not necessarily apply to individuals. The population asymptote implies that the age at which a cohort becomes sterile is indetermi- nate, but claims of maternity after the sixth decade are not well documented. The record for late maternity is presently held by Ruth Alice Kistler, an American woman, who gave birth to a daughter in 1956 at the age of 57 years and 129 days (Fergusson et al., 1982). During the span of fertile ages the secondary sex ratio is fairly stable, tending to fall slightly with increased parental age (Russell, 1936; Garfinkel and Selvin, 1976).

Some of the most reliable estimates of natural fertility in married couples have been obtained from Hutterite communities in North America (Eaton and Mayer, 1953). The Hutterites are members of an Anabaptist sect who emigrated in the nineteenth century to escape religious persecution in Europe. Their beliefs strict- ly prohibit contraception, abortion and extra-marital coitus. The lack of any artificial restraints on fertility within the marital bond combined with a short duration of lactation and high standards of diet, housing and medical care have produced some of the highest fertility rates on record. These rates are close to the theoretical maximum, though presently falling as elsewhere in North America (Laing, 1980). The distribution of live births among Hutterites is far less skewed than it is in the American population as a whole because of greater fertility

TABLE 5.2

Fertility among the Ethnic Hutterites: Age-Specific Fertility Rates[a] and Percentage of Sterile Couples by Age Group[b]

Age of the mother (years)	Annual number of live births per 1000 women	Sterile couples at end of age interval (%)
15–19	12.0	3.5
20–24	231.0	
25–29	382.7	7
30–34	391.1	11
35–39	344.6	33
40–44	208.3	87
45–49	42.1	100
15–49	226.6	—

[a] Reprinted from *Human Biology,* Vol. 25, No. 3 (1953), by Joseph W. Eaton and Albert J. Mayer by permission of the Wayne State University Press. Copyright (1953) by the Wayne State University Press.

[b] From Tietze, C. (1957). Reproductive span and rate of reproduction among Hutterite women. *Fertil. Steril.* **8**, 89. Reproduced with permission of the publisher, The American Fertility Society.

among older cohorts and because early marriage is discouraged (Table 5.2). The birth rate of Hutterites fell after the third decade of maternal age, and between ages 35 and 49 the percentage of women who ceased to reproduce rose from 10 to 100%. The average age at last confinement was 40.9 years, in accord with findings from other populations. The interval between confinements was surprisingly constant throughout reproductive life, apart from substantially longer intervals between the final two pregnancies. It must be remembered that these data show the natural fertility of married couples, and the contributions of male infertility and reduced coital rates are not recognizable. Such limitations have been overcome using records from programmes of artificial insemination by donor (AID) in which the male factor is uniquely controlled.

A large-scale survey of experience with AID in France has shown that female fecundity begins to fail at about the mid-point of menstrual life (Fédération CECOS *et al.*, 1982). The subjects were presumed to be fecund on the basis of azoospermia of their husbands and the absence of gynaecological disease. The time taken for 50% of them to achieve a clinically recognizable pregnancy after joining the programme was 6 months for those aged less than 30, 7 months for those aged 31–35 and >12 months for older women (Fig. 5.1). These interesting results imply that fecundity begins to fall a few years before the age when menstrual cycles are most regular (see Section 4.3). They also have clear implications for women who wish to defer reproduction, but it should be emphasized that the prognosis for fertility in the fourth decade is still relatively good

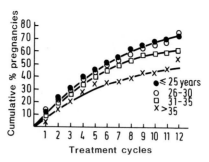

Fig. 5.1. Cumulative success rates of human artificial insemination cycles for four maternal age ranges. The rates for the two youngest age ranges (<26 and 26–30 years) are represented by a single tracing because they are similar. These rates were significantly higher than for older women aged 31–35 ($P < .03$) and >35 years ($P < .001$). (From Fédération CECOS et al., 1982; reprinted by permission of the *New England Journal of Medicine* **306**, 404–406.)

and the outcome of pregnancy is satisfactory in most cases (Bongaarts, 1982). Natural sexual unions are generally more successful than AID since sperm are damaged during freezing and thawing and the fertile time of the cycle may be missed. In the CECOS study only 0.1 successful conceptions were obtained on average per woman per month, whereas natural insemination is often twice as successful and may even reach 0.4–0.5 in optimally fertile couples when coitus occurs daily (Schwartz et al., 1980). Nevertheless, the CECOS study is of considerable interest, and biologists must now seek to explain the early loss of fecundity in our own species.

5.3. Biological Basis of Infertility in Middle Age

Occurrence of Fetal Wastage

In middle-aged rodents, the litter size falls in advance of a significant reduction in the number of corpora lutea (Jones, 1970). Although a larger proportion of ovulatory follicles fail to liberate their ova, the number of these faults is relatively small, and so the loss of fertility is attributable mainly to postovulatory failure (R. G. Gosden, unpublished observations). Most of the infertility arises from intra-uterine mortality of implanted fetuses, and in C57BL/6J mice, the death rate peaks after mid-gestation (day 10) when the allantois assumes primary responsibility for placentation (Fig. 5.2). Since dead fetuses are soft and macerated and cannot be evacuated from uterine horns in polytocous species without disturbing viable siblings, they are eliminated by resorption *in utero*, being reduced to a dark spot or "mole" by full term. There are statistical grounds for suspecting that when an entire litter is aborted systemic factors are

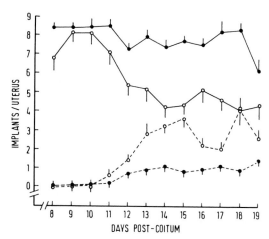

Fig. 5.2. Variation in the number of live (—) and resorbing fetuses (_ _ _) in C57BL/6J mice aged 3–7 (●) or 11–12 months (○). Pregnancy dates begin on the day of mating (day 1). Values given are means ± SEM. (Redrawn from the data of Holinka *et al.*, 1979, and Gosden *et al.*, 1981; reprinted with permission.)

responsible, whereas individual fetal death occurs sporadically in the uterus, which is perhaps a reflection of local deterioration of the environment (Gosden *et al.*, 1981). Some conceptuses are lost at other stages of gestation, particularly the transitional stages of fertilization, implantation and parturition (Blaha, 1964; Fabricant *et al.*, 1978; Holinka *et al.*, 1978; Mizoguchi and Dukelow, 1981).

Approximately 10–15% of all clinically recognizable pregnancies in women who are apparently fertile terminate spontaneously by abortion. Such figures underestimate the global proportion lost, which has been estimated to be as high as 78% (Roberts and Lowe, 1975). The extent of embryonic and fetal losses can now be estimated prospectively from an early postimplantation age by measuring the specific β subunit of hCG in urine (Miller *et al.*, 1980). In a study of healthy, sexually active women, 62% of conceptuses detected by this method were lost by 12 weeks of gestation (Edmonds *et al.*, 1982). Many of those lost were recognized only by a transient elevation of hCG. That human embryos are frequently lost at early stages, including preimplantation, was indicated by morphological studies of Hertig *et al.* (1959), who observed that 10 out of 34 embryos were abnormal during the first 2 weeks after conception. Some of these embryos are likely to have been chromosomally imbalanced, judging by preliminary results with *in vitro* fertilization (Angell *et al.*, 1983). However, despite this progress, it is not yet possible to confidently estimate the total extent of pregnancy failure in normal women, and it is even more difficult to gauge the effects of ageing.

The incidence of spontaneous abortion in women rises with age (Fig. 5.3). Parity (birth order) might be an independent risk factor (Naylor and Warburton,

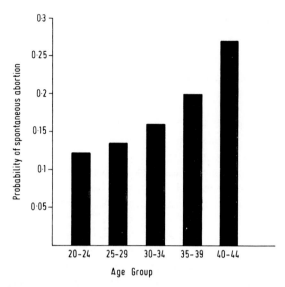

Fig. 5.3.   Variation in the rate of human spontaneous abortion according to maternal age (overall mean rate, 150/1000). (From Leridon, ''Human Fertility. The Basic Components.'' © 1977 by The University of Chicago. Reprinted with permission.)

1979). However, the probability of abortion for any given individual does not necessarily increase year by year as the survey data suggest. The relationship between age and abortion rate could be a statistical artefact of reproductive compensation (James, 1974a). For example, Aberdeen women with successful pregnancy histories restricted their reproductive activity during the fourth and fifth decades to a greater extent than abortion-prone women, who were then over-represented in these age groups (Billewicz, 1973). The artefact hypothesis predicts that the relationship between abortion incidence and maternal age (or parity) would be less marked in societies that encourage large families. Confirmatory evidence has been obtained from the Amish community in the United States (Resseguie, 1974), details of pregnancy wastage in Hutterite women being lacking at the present time. Nevertheless, it is probable that the rising incidence of fetal death is partly owing to biological effects of maternal age. Records from an *in vitro* fertilization and embryo transfer programme indicate that a large proportion of conceptuses are lost near the time of implantation. Between 15 and 21% of embryos conceived extra-corporeally implanted successfully in native mothers aged 20–39, whereas only 0–7% did so in older women (Edwards and Steptoe, 1983). Conceptuses in older mothers might be at greater risk at all stages of gestation, although it is most likely that transitional stages in development are most hazardous, as in animals. Those that survive gestation in mothers aged >39 are also more likely to die during the perinatal period (Naeye, 1983), but social factors contribute to this increased risk, as in the case of higher mortality rates among women of high parity (Department of Health and Social Security, 1982).

Errors of Oogenesis and Embryo Development

Chromosomal Anomalies

Chromosomally defective fetuses form a large portion of human reproductive wastage at all ages. Cytogenetic surveys in several parts of the world and among different racial groups show that about 50% of all spontaneous abortuses of the first trimester are chromosomally aberrant, a smaller percentage being found at later stages of gestation (reviewed by Bond and Chandley, 1983). Since 10–15% of all clinically recognizable pregnancies terminate in abortion, a minimum of 5–10% of conceptuses are chromosomally imperfect in man. It is not yet clear whether sub-human primates have such a remarkably high incidence of anomalies, but in rodents the figures are almost an order of magnitude lower. The frequencies of various abnormal karyotypes among early abortuses have a characteristic pattern, as is illustrated by data obtained in France (Boué et al., 1975). In that survey, autosomal trisomy accounted for 52% of the anomalies recorded. All chromosome groups (A–G) were involved, though anomalies of the larger chromosomal groups, A and B, were proportionately under-represented. Only 15% of the anomalies were monosomies, most of these being 45,XO (potentially Turner's syndrome). If aneuploidy arises only from non-disjunction and each chromosome pair affected migrates randomly to either pole of the spindle, trisomic and monosomic fetuses would be conceived in equal numbers. In fact, monosomy can arise also by failure of a single chromosome to be transported from the equator of the spindle ("anaphase lagging"). The observed lower frequencies of monosomies are not inconsistent with theory if these die at very early stages of gestation, as they do in experimental animal models (Gropp, 1976). The other major group of anomalies in the French survey was triploidy, comprising 20% of the total; the remaining groups included small numbers of fetuses with tetraploidy or structural defects of the karyotype.

Fortunately, the majority of chromosomally anomalous fetuses conceived are not well adapted to life in utero, and the incidence of chromosomal aberration in full-term babies is less than 1% at most maternal ages (Hook, 1981). The survivors are mainly trisomies of small chromosomes, yet even these are only a small proportion of the number conceived. The causes of prenatal death are poorly understood. In the case of monosomy, the absence of essential "housekeeping" genes carried by X chromosomes or autosomes can explain early embryonic death. In trisomy the effects of chromosomal imbalance are generally less severe, especially if sex chromosomes are involved; nevertheless, trisomy is invariably associated with some form of phenotypic disturbance with retarded growth of both embryonic and extra-embryonic tissue (Mittwoch and Delhanty,

1972; Gropp, 1976; Honoré *et al.,* 1976). Eventually, the teratogenic effects of chromosomal imbalance will be explained by gene mapping and developmental biology. There are some indications already that the additional gene dosage is fully expressed in chromosomally aberrant cells. In erythrocytes and fibroblasts of Down's syndrome patients (trisomy 21) there is 50% excess activity of two enzymes specified by chromosome 21, namely, superoxide dismutase-1 and phosphoribosylglycinamide sythetase (see Epstein *et al.,* 1982). Failure to suppress supernumerary genes responsible for these products may not be serious, but if this applies to genes responsible for membrane proteins, there are likely to be implications for cellular interactions, growth and migration. Such effects could be responsible for abnormal phenotypes and death through failure of a critical organ or simply by growth retardation (Polani, 1974).

The incidence of several clinically significant chromosome disorders in newborn babies rises with maternal age. The distribution is J-shaped for some disorders because of a small excess in incidence amongst newborns of teenage mothers compared with newborns of slightly older mothers (Smith and Berg, 1976; Erickson, 1978; Hook, 1981). In an American survey, 0.2% of neonates born to mothers less than 30 years old were chromosomally abnormal, but the incidence rose to 1.6% for those aged 40 and to 5.4% for 45-year-old mothers (Fig. 5.4). The most common anomaly among older mothers, Down's syndrome, has been known to be associated with maternal age for more than a century. The incidence of trisomy of the following chromosomes rises at similar rates from different baselines: chromosome numbers 13 and 18 and X (Court Brown *et al.,* 1969; Hook, 1981). A maternal age relationship has been found amongst most trisomic abortuses (with the exception of trisomy 16) but not for monosomy X, triploidy or mosaic karyotypes. Penrose (1933, 1961) demonstrated that Down's syndrome in babies was related to maternal age rather than to paternal age or parity. Furthermore, since the maternal age distributions were bimodal in some samples, he proposed that they represent the superposition of two distinct Gaussian distributions, one of which has characteristics similar to those of mothers of normal infants (class A), with the other representing the higher incidence among late maternities (class B). The mean age of mothers in class B is about 38, 10 years greater than A. Down's babies in class A, which is independent of age, arise either *de novo* from environmental factors or from hereditary causes such as structural translocations and parental aneuploidy, whether total or mosaic. Those in class B are usually more abundant (c. 60%), as depicted in the distribution for abortuses (Fig. 5.5). The risk of delivering a Down's baby rises three- to fourfold every 5 years after age 30, although some data show the rate of ascent is less steep during the final years of fertile life (Collmann and Stoller, 1962; Hook, 1981). Such irregularities of the age distribution have obstructed attempts to fit equations, which would have theoretical implications for understanding the aetiology of trisomy. A simple exponential

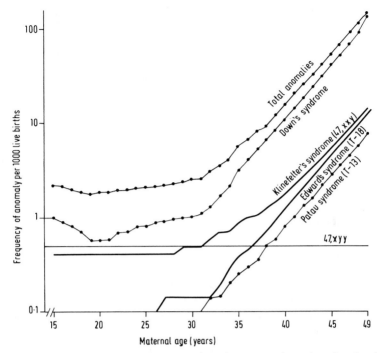

Fig. 5.4.   Incidence of trisomy of autosomes and sex chromosomes in newborn American babies according to maternal age. (Adapted from Hook, 1981. Reprinted with permission from The American College of Obstetricians and Gynecologists. *Obstet. Gynecol.* **58**, 282–285).

function would indicate that a series of independent or accidental events is responsible for trisomy, but such a curve is only a rough approximation to the data. The discontinuous form of the age distribution has been attributed to statistical artefacts (reproductive compensation or limitation among mothers of affected children), interactions of age with environmental risk factors and increased fetal mortality in older mothers, but these require further study.

The reduction divisions of meiosis responsible for trisomy 21 have now been identified using stains which produce specific and reproducible banding patterns on human chromosomes. The use of chromosomal heteromorphisms for tracing the origin of supernumerary chromosomes depends on Mendelian principles of segregation and can be illustrated by the following simple example. In an informative mating in which four chromosomal variants are present, designated ab in the father and cd in the mother, a trisomic child with acd or bcd will have arisen by chromosomal non-disjunction at metaphase I in the mother. If the child had any of the combinations aac/aad/bbc/bbd, a fault at metaphase II in the father must have been responsible. By using such methods it has been possible to show that the majority of human trisomies originate, irrespective of maternal age, at

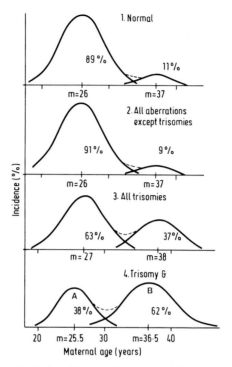

Fig. 5.5.   Percentage distribution of human abortuses according to maternal age (see text for description). Panel 1: normal karyotype. Panel 2: monosomy X, triploidy, tetraploidy and structural anomalies of the karyotype. Panel 3: all trisomies. Panel 4: trisomy G, showing class A (independent of maternal age) and class B (dependent on age). M, mean age. (From Boué *et al.*, 1975; reprinted with permission).

the first meiotic division of oocytes (Jacobs and Hassold, 1980; Mikkelsen *et al.*, 1980). They also demonstrate that most triploid fetuses arise by dispermic fertilization (Jacobs *et al.*, 1978; Lauritsen *et al.*, 1979). However, the male is not exonerated from responsibility for aneuploid offspring because these have sometimes been traced to errors in spermatocytes. Direct examination of human spermatozoal karyotypes is not possible on a large scale, except by allowing penetration of hamster ova following removal of the zona pellucida. This method has shown that 5% of human spermatozoa are aneusomic (Martin *et al.*, 1983), and it is expected that it will soon help to extend knowledge of paternal ageing. This may help to clarify the results of epidemiological studies, which are almost equally divided between those showing a slight positive effect of paternal age and those in which aneuploidy was independent of this factor (Roecker and Huether, 1983).

The incidence of trisomy at full term is the product of two probabilities:

chromosomal non-disjunction and survival *in utero*. It has been suggested that the incidence rises because of relaxed selection against anomalous fetuses in older mothers (Aymé and Lippman-Hand, 1982). This conclusion is not accepted by a number of authorities (Carothers, 1983; Hook, 1983; Warburton *et al.*, 1983) and is at variance with the observed higher frequency in spontaneous abortuses (see Fig. 5.5) (Alberman *et al.*, 1976; Hassold *et al.*, 1980) and higher incidence of aneuploidy among zygotes and preimplantation embryos in older mice (see Bond and Chandley, 1983). Despite this latter finding, fewer abnormal pups are delivered at full term (Parsons, 1964; Goodlin, 1965). This situation might arise from competition between abnormal fetuses and their more vigorous siblings for some limited resource, such as the blood supply, in the compromising environment of older uteri.

The increase of trisomy in long-lived oocytes has sometimes been attributed to accumulated damage inflicted by agencies in the external environment. The smaller (if present) effect of paternal age could be explained by natural selection of the normal, more vigorous cells in the continuously proliferating male germ line. Although the loss of microtubules could lead to chromosomal non-disjunction by failing to provide a balance between the traction forces in the meiotic spindle, ageing effects must be indirect because the spindle is not assembled until shortly before the reduction division. It has been suggested that older oocytes are more vulnerable to ionizing radiation and chemical mutagens, but studies could not confirm this hypothesis (Tease, 1982; Golbus, 1983). Other environmental factors have been imputed, namely, atmospheric pollution, thyroid autoimmunity, fluoride in drinking water supplies, viral hepatitis (see Smith and Berg, 1976; Bond and Chandley, 1983) and, most recently, smoking (Kline *et al.*, 1983). But the worldwide distribution of Down's syndrome would seem to deny that environmental variables have a primary role, although they might explain temporal and geographic fluctuations in frequency (Collmann and Stoller, 1962; Evans *et al.*, 1978; Read, 1982). In recent years, workers have increasingly concentrated their search for an explanation of age-dependent trisomy on internal factors.

Postovulatory deterioration of oocytes is one of the factors which has been considered. Zygotes are more frequently triploid or carry other abnormal features if fertilized after the short span of optimal ripeness (Austin, 1970). Since there is no oestrous phase at mid-cycle to synchronize human ovulation and insemination, German (1968) postulated that the risk of conceiving a Down's zygote would increase with age because the probability of delayed fertilization is greater in older women who engage in coitus less frequently. The mechanism of aneuploidy has then been explained either by premature disjunction of chromatids in over-ripened oocytes (Rodman, 1971) or by failure of a chromosome in a sub-nucleus of a zygote to unite with those on the metaphase plate of the first cleavage division (Austin, 1970). However, German's hypothesis has not been substantiated statistically (Cannings and Cannings, 1968), nor is it compatible with the evidence that most chromosomal non-disjunction occurs before ovulation during the first reduction division.

Alternatively, it has been proposed that oocytes are qualitatively inferior when shed from follicles after a prolonged follicular phase (Hertig, 1967; Jongbloet, 1975). This hypothesis is not easily reconciled with the observed reduction in the length of this phase in ageing women (p. 73). Furthermore, phase length was not a factor for the fertility of women joining an AID programme, although the number of women with follicular phases <12 and >17 days long is admittedly small (Broom *et al.*, 1981). This hypothesis is, however, corroborated by a rising incidence of developmental anomalies and chromosomal imbalance following delayed ovulation in the toad, *Xenopus laevis* (Mikamo, 1968). It is much more difficult to test whether comparable effects of intra-follicular ageing occur in laboratory mammals because ova are more scarce and aneuploidy is comparatively rare. In these animals, ovulation can be delayed by inhibiting the release of ovulatory amounts of gonadotrophins using either barbiturates (Butcher and Fugo, 1967; Mikamo and Hamaguchi, 1975) or antibodies raised against LHRH (Laing *et al.*, 1984). The maximum extension of Graafian follicle life is limited by atresia, which afflicts most follicles on the third day postoestrus. No statistically significant increase in trisomy has been obtained using these methods. Since only trisomy is associated with maternal ageing, the greater abundance of triploid and mosaic embryos after delaying ovulation with barbiturates indicates that cycle length extension has different effects from those of ageing.

According to Henderson and Edwards (1968), trisomy may arise at the first reduction division from random segregation of univalents formed by inadequate bonding of chromosome pairs established prenatally during oogenesis. Their hypothesis is based on an inverse relationship between maternal age and chiasma frequency in oocytes, which has been confirmed in several laboratories (Polani and Jagiello, 1976; Luthardt *et al.*, 1973; Speed, 1977; Sugawara and Mikamo, 1983). Since chiasmata are formed during oogenesis, Henderson and Edwards proposed that there is a programmed sequence of utilization of oocytes in which those formed first are ovulated first, and so on. Since oogenesis continues over many weeks in primates (Peters, 1970), it is possible that changing conditions of the internal environment affect oocytes; even in mice, in which this process is brief, germ cells proceed asynchronously through meiosis (Dietrich and Mulder, 1983). For technical reasons it has been difficult to verify this ''production line'' hypothesis either by labelling premeiotic germ cells with radiolabelled nucleosides or by estimating the recombination frequency for linked genes. To confirm the hypothesis, this frequency should fall *pari passu* with chiasma frequency. This hypothesis, once widely held, is now receiving more critical appraisal. In Chinese hamsters there was little correspondence between the chromosome groups involved in univalent formation at metaphase I and those responsible for aneuploidy at the ensuing maturation division (Sugawara and Mikamo,

1983). Furthermore, despite a careful search, no gradient of chromosome anomalies among oocytes exists at successive stages of oogenesis (Speed and Chandley, 1983). A final verdict cannot be passed yet on whether chromosome anomalies are preformed in the fetal ovary. If they are not, some hope remains for eventually controlling their production later in life.

Some evidence suggests that trisomy should be seen within the setting of the wider physiological changes of the ageing female. This hypothesis is less discrete than those mentioned so far, but there is some experimental support for suspecting that ageing of oocytes is an epiphenomenon of the general deterioration of the reproductive system. Brook *et al.* (1984) reported that in unilaterally ovariectomized mice, the rising incidence of aneuploid embryos during ageing began earlier and cyclical ovarian function terminated earlier than in controls. These results suggest that the risk of non-disjunction in oocytes is increased during the final cycles of life, irrespective of the chronological age of the mother. According to some workers, it is the prolongation of these cycles that is significant because spontaneous or drug-induced extension of cycle length in rats leads to more morphologically abnormal embryos (Fugo and Butcher, 1971; Page *et al.*, 1983). However, in view of what has been said already about delayed ovulation, it is unlikely that longer cycles are wholly to blame for trisomy. Since the incidence of human trisomies in the population rises long before the irregular cycles of the climacteric, the possibility of subtle hormonal changes affecting follicular oocytes is worth considering. Ovarian steroids can impair segregation of meiotic chromosomes during maturation *in vitro* (McGaughey, 1977), and a case has been made for hormone-dependent changes in the timing of maturation leading to trisomy (Crowley *et al.*, 1979). These views can accommodate the J-shaped age distribution for trisomy because ovarian cycles are more irregular at both ends of the menstrual span (see p. 72). Changes in the frequency of Down's syndrome among young women have also been attributed to altered hormonal balance following oral contraception (Read, 1982). To extend the argument to a logical conclusion, any factor that advances the normal course of ovarian ageing and its associated hormonal changes might potentiate the increase in trisomy. This would then explain the excess of trisomic offspring among smokers (Kline *et al.*, 1983) and among Turner's syndrome patients, in whom pregnancy is sometimes possible before early menopause (Reyes *et al.*, 1976; King *et al.*, 1978). However, we should not be sanguine about untested hypotheses, especially when an earlier study was unable to demonstrate an association between Down's syndrome and less regular menses or early menopause in mothers (Sigler *et al.*, 1967). The maternal age factor is still one of the major unsolved problems of human cytogenetics.

Other Anomalies of Development

Germ cells are segregated from somatic cells at early stages of embryogenesis, and some of their descendants survive for most, if not all, of the lifespan. For much of this span they are not multiplying, and natural selection cannot operate to maintain vigour in the population. Yet, apart from those becoming chromosomally imbalanced, their progeny after fertilization have the same fertile potential and longevity as the parents. Furthermore, epidemiological studies have found little evidence that germ cells accumulate fresh gene mutations during ageing, and the effects that have been found are attributed mainly to paternal age (Polednak, 1976; Roberts, 1979). The ability of germ cells to avoid the costs of ageing, which are manifest among somatic cells, has fascinated biologists for generations. Germ cells which succeed in producing progeny are presumably either peculiarly resistant to damage of their informational macromolecules or have highly efficient repair mechanisms, which perhaps involve events during meiosis (Medvedev, 1981). This special quality of germ cells applies to most species, including mammals (Suntzeff et al., 1962), a notable exception being the "Lansing effect" of the freshwater rotifer *Philodina citrina*. Eggs from ageing clones of this species become progressively less viable and new individuals arising from them become precociously senile, but this phenomenon seems to be confined to the parthenogenetic mode of reproduction in these simple animals (Lansing, 1947).

Finally, mention should be made of human neural tube defects, for although they probably arise from a vitamin deficiency or an environmental agency, rather than being a general feature of ageing, their incidence varies during maternal ageing with a U-shaped distribution. Above age 35, the incidence of spina bifida and anencephalus is independent of parity, as is the age-related increase of hydrocephalus (Record, 1961; Carter et al., 1968; Carter and Evans, 1973). Further study is required to discover whether the age factor is due to variable penetrance by the causal agent or to differential viability in utero.

The Maternal Environment

Changes with Age

Increased pregnancy loss in ageing animals cannot be accounted for by defective embryos alone. The balance of responsibility between the maternal environment on the one hand and embryonic factors on the other has been shown by transferring zygotes or preimplantation embryos from young to old animals and vice versa. In small rodents it is necessary first to make the hosts pseudopregnant by mating with a vasectomized male because the corpora lutea are not active spontaneously during normal oestrous cycles. Results have shown unequivocally that animals of middle or old age perform poorly, for less than 15% of embryos from young donors were successful in older hosts, whereas approximately 50% survived to term in hosts of similar age (Table 5.3). In the experiments shown in Table 5.3, and in subsequent confirmatory ones, embryonic losses were found at both pre- and postimplantation stages.

TABLE 5.3

Relative Contributions of Embryonic and Maternal Factors in the Loss of Fertility during Ageing: Comparison of Three Species Using Reciprocal Transfer of Embryos between Young and Ageing Animals

		Embryos surviving to term (%)		
Age of donor	Age of host	Hamster[a]	Rabbit[b]	Mouse[c]
Young	Young	49	50	48
Young	Old	8	2	14
Old	Young	5	13	54

[a] Blaha (1964).
[b] Adams (1970).
[c] Talbert and Krohn (1966).

It has been suggested that embryos may be dying at the time of implantation because the normal development schedule of the embryo and endometrium are desynchronized. This state of affairs could arise from a reduced rate of cleavage, which has been observed in old hamsters (Parkening and Soderwall, 1973). However, this would not appear to be the principal factor because transfer of preimplantation embryos which are one day in advance of the development of the ageing host uterus does not subsequently improve pregnancy success. The time taken for transporting embryos along the oviduct is about 3 days in both young and ageing mothers, but obstruction of the channel by stones could affect fertility in some species (Adams, 1970), although ectopic pregnancy in the oviduct is most exceptional in animals of any age (Gosden and Russell, 1981).

At the time of implantation, the uterine epithelium is thrown into folds which probably support blastocysts during the transport and attachment phases. This support is impaired in ageing rodents in which luminal epithelia fail to undergo corrugation changes and engage one another (Finn, 1970). Furthermore, attachment of trophectoderm cells of the blastocyst to the uterine epithelium may be hindered because microvilli on the surfaces of the latter are morphologically abnormal (Smith, 1975) or sparse (see Fig. 5.6). That this deficiency is not dependent on the systemic environment has been shown by the failure of uterine epithelia of 6- and 30-month-old CBA mice to adopt the appearance of the host following transplantation between different age groups (Fig. 5.6). In apparent contrast, it has been suggested that steroid treatment of the human postmenopausal endometrium restores the normal morphology of epithelial surfaces (Nathan *et al.*, 1978).

Preparation for and maintenance of postimplantation development depend on stimulation by oestrogen and progesterone (Psychoyos, 1973). Blood levels of these hormones have been compared in many studies of ageing rodents, and most

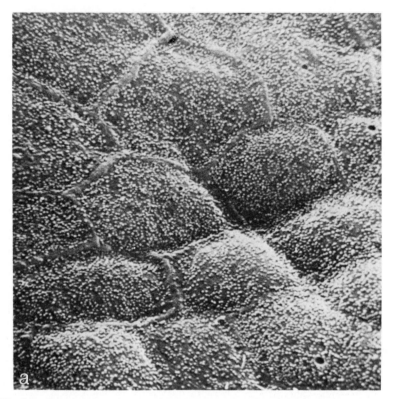

Fig. 5.6. Scanning electron micrographs of the luminal surface of uteri of CBA mice, showing a greater density of microvilli in (a) a young uterine graft in an old host compared with (b) an old uterine graft in a young host (X10,000). (From the late E. C. Jones, unpublished.)

results show that neither hormone is deficient (Spilman *et al.*, 1972; Gosden and Fowler, 1979; Holinka *et al.*, i979; Miller and Riegle, 1980). Although corpora lutea form and function normally in these animals, those of cows tend to become cystic, leading to infertility late in the second decade of life (Erickson *et al.*, 1976). It is important to consider whether hormonal changes preceding conception are altered by ageing because uterine receptivity depends on an appropriate strength, duration and sequence of stimulation by gonadal steroids (Finn and Martin, 1970). In middle-aged rats, the uterus is exposed to oestrogen for a longer period, corresponding to the extension of cycle length at this phase (Page and Butcher, 1982), and this condition has been held responsible for some of the subsequent embryonic mortality (Butcher and Pope, 1979; Page *et al.*, 1983).

In climacteric women, menstrual cycles are often infertile owing to luteolysis within 10 days of ovulation (Table 4.1). A short luteal phase is likely to be of greater significance for fertility than are relatively small reductions in peak

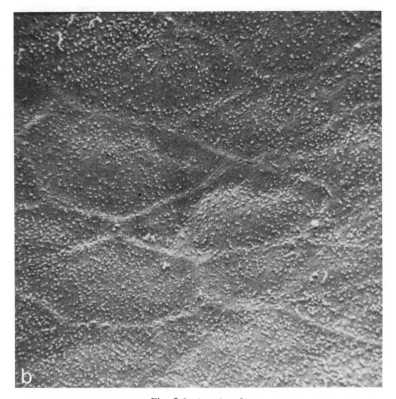

Fig. 5.6. (*continued*)

amounts of progesterone in middle-aged women (Reyes *et al.*, 1977) because an embryo may be unable to rescue the corpus luteum, and so perishes. In contrast to the situation in laboratory rodents, responsibility for producing most of the gestational steroids in human pregnancy is progressively transferred from the ovary to the placenta, which assumes primary responsibility at about 6 weeks of gestation (Csapo *et al.*, 1974). It would be interesting to have more information about the function of the feto-placental unit in older mothers, in view of the higher incidence of large placental infarcts and other placental disorders in women over 40, especially among smokers (Naeye, 1979).

Following the demonstration of normal luteal activity in most ageing animals, attention was diverted to the measurement of hormone-binding capacity in target tissues in order to find alternative explanations for poor adaptation of the uterus to gestation. Most evidence obtained from human and rodent uteri suggests that neither concentrations nor physical characteristics of cytosolic receptors for oestrogen and progesterone are affected by ageing (Flickinger *et al.*, 1977; Blaha and Leavitt, 1978; Belisle *et al.*, 1982); discrepant results were obtained only with animals of postreproductive age (Gesell and Roth, 1981). One study shows that a significant fraction of the oestrogen–receptor complexes in the postmenopausal uterus are unable to bind to nuclear acceptor sites and are therefore biologically inactive (Strathy *et al.*, 1982). This result is probably secondary to a changing endocrine milieu, for there can be no doubt that the human endometrium is capable of responding to ovarian steroids long after menopause and that normal uterotrophic responses can be obtained in animals of advanced age (Holinka *et al.*, 1977). Pregnancies are occasionally reported in middle-aged women after menopause, as conventionally defined, but these are invariably unsuccessful (Krohn, 1964). A well-documented case has now been described in a woman aged only 25 who had menopause of at least 5 years' standing (Lutjen *et al.*, 1984). After several attempts, an embryo derived by fertilization *in vitro* of a donor's egg with her husband's spermatozoon was successfully brought to term with the support of exogenous hormones. Similarly, the uterus of CBA mice of postreproductive age is occasionally capable of maintaining gestation when stimulated by ovarian grafts, confirming that atrophic changes can be reversed (Krohn, 1964; Felicio *et al.*, 1984).

In ageing uteri, several notable cytological changes occur which could contribute to postimplantation death. Considerable attention has been focussed on the decidual cell reaction, not because any definite function can yet be assigned to it but because it is dramatically reduced (Finn, 1966; Maibenco and Krehbiel, 1973; Holinka and Finch, 1977). The reaction may be impaired because production of prostaglandin (particularly PGE-2) is reduced (Brown *et al.*, 1984), this group of substances having been implicated in early postimplantation physiology, including hyperaemia and decidualization (Tobert, 1976; Kennedy, 1977).

Surprisingly little attention has been paid to the possibility that postimplantation conceptuses die because of inadequate vascular perfusion. It is well known that when blood flow to the placenta is restricted by ligating uterine vessels, fetal development is retarded, sometimes leading to resorption (Wigglesworth, 1964). During ageing in rabbits the rate of blood flow to the gravid uterus is halved when calculated per unit weight of tissue (Larson and Foote, 1972). This result could simply be due to lower respiratory demands, and so measurements of lactate and blood gases in uterine veins are needed to check this finding. These measurements of uterine blood flow also highlight a problem which is frequently encountered when comparing young and ageing tissues which have differing compositions. The greater proportion of collagen in old tissues leads to an underestimate of cellular perfusion when unit weights of tissue are compared. Underperfusion of placentas in old uteri would be expected to lead to smaller fetal size, but newborn pups are of normal weight for litter size (R. G. Gosden, unpublished observations), and in our own species birth weight increases with parity (Selvin and Janerich, 1971). The sclerotic changes which cause stenosis of uterine vessels in multiparous rodents and women (Wexler, 1964; Naeye, 1983) may be of little consequence if there are compensatory changes involving more efficient oxygen extraction in the placenta or, in polytocous species, if death of some fetuses releases resources for remaining ones. Nevertheless, it seems prudent for older mothers to rest, control any hypertension and refrain from smoking in order to optimize the utero-placental circulation.

The ageing uterus of rodents steadily accumulates collagen (Schaub, 1964–1965), whereas the collagen content of human uteri has been found to be constant between 30 years of age and menopause (Woessner, 1963). The accumula-

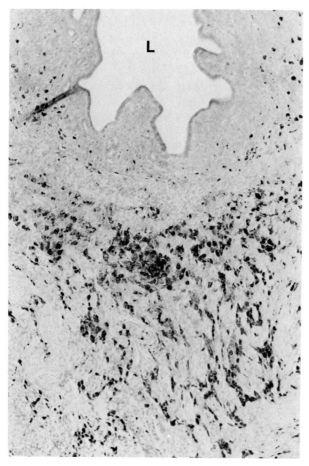

Fig. 5.7. Transverse section of the uterine wall of a multiparous mouse, showing abundant phagocytes laden with haemosiderin in the muscle coat of the mesometrial side. L, lumen. Perl's stain and neutral red (X75). (From Gosden, 1979.)

tion of fibre can be attributed to less catabolism because of (1) greater physical and chemical stability conferred by covalent intermolecular bonding (Kao *et al.*, 1976) and (2) less collagenase (Maurer and Foote, 1972). These changes could be adaptive, though most workers suspect that they lead to detrimental changes, perhaps affecting the compliance of the uterus and cervix during gestation and parturition.

Scar tissue accumulating at former sites of placentation is another factor which might affect subsequent implantations. It consists of macrophages replete with lipofuscin and haemosiderin pigments which are residues of "mopping-up" operations *postpartum* (Fig. 5.7). These pigments are responsible for the yellow-brown coloration of multiparous rodent uteri and should not be confused with vitamin E deficiency pigments, which have similar histochemical properties but are found in uterine smooth muscle cells. Vitamin E deficiency leads to dystrophy of uterine muscle and fetal death in rats (Kitabchi, 1980), but there is no general evidence, from either histochemistry or vitamin supplementation work, to show a deficiency during ageing, despite one claim that vitamin E requirements rise steeply with age (Ames, 1974). The most conspicuous cytological change affecting the human uterus is the accumulation of autofluorescent particles beginning at the time of puberty (Fig. 5.8). Though they are abundant by middle age, the significance of these particles is obscure.

Effects of Reproductive History

Since pregnancy and lactation impose enormous metabolic demands, high parity might be expected to cause adverse wear and tear on the maternal constitution and perhaps accentuate specific pathophysiological changes, such as sclerosis of blood vessel walls. This assumption is difficult to verify in our own species because superabundant reproduction is commonly associated with social deprivation and poor standards of obstetric care, diet and housing. At the opposite end of the spectrum of reproductive output, primigravidae aged more than 34 years take longer to establish a successful pregnancy (Guttmacher, 1956) and have a high age-specific rate of perinatal mortality (Israel and Deutschberger, 1964). Such findings ought not to be accepted uncritically as a biological effect because this group may be self-selected for poor fertility following earlier unsuccessful attempts to reproduce (see p. 98). This limitation on the interpretation of human fertility statistics can be avoided by studying animals for which some definite biological effects of parity have been found under the special conditions of intra-uterine fetal crowding.

First, it is necessary to emphasize that no simple wear and tear hypothesis can accommodate all the facts concerning ageing and litter size because animals are not protected from the normal age-dependent toll of fetal death when mating is delayed until mid-life. According to some studies, elderly primigravid rats and mice are rather less fertile than multiparous animals of similar age (Asdell *et al.*,

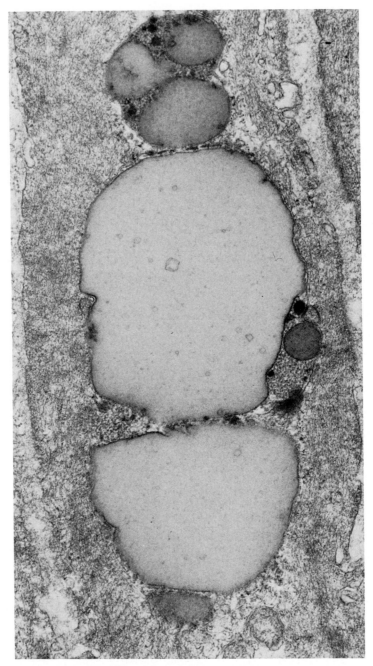

Fig. 5.8. Uterine smooth muscle cell from a 48-year-old multiparous woman. The cell contains membrane-bound particles of variable electron density, with satellite dense bodies (presumably lysosomes). Osmium tetroxide (X47,200). (From Gosden *et al.*, 1978.)

1941; Nishimura and Shikata, 1960). The effects of parity have been tested experimentally in rodents following unilateral ovariectomy at young adult ages. The remaining ovary sheds double its normal quota of ova, which, if fertilized, will implant only in tbe ipsilateral uterine horn. Thus, one of each pair of horns carries double the normal load of fetuses, whereas the other one remains barren, though subject to the same systemic hormonal conditions. The total number of live offspring produced after unilateral ovariectomy was approximately halved compared with that of intact controls, though there were detailed differences in breeding patterns according to the rodent species tested (Jones and Krohn, 1960; Biggers *et al.*, 1962; Adams, 1970). In rats, litter size fell sharply after the sixth delivery, though not to zero, as in some strains of mice (Fig. 5.9), whereas in rabbits it declined steadily throughout life (Adams, 1970). Since corpora lutea and conceptuses were still produced after delivery of the final litter, Biggers *et al.* (1962) postulated that accelerated uterine ageing of the functional horn was responsible for pregnancy failure. Confirmation was obtained when it was found

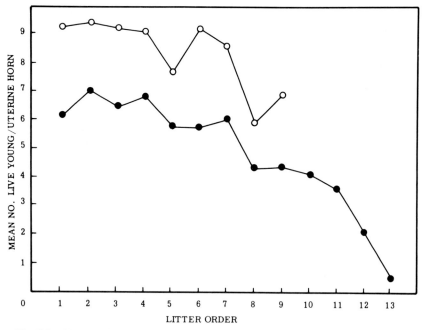

Fig. 5.9.   Mean number of live young produced per functional uterine horn during the lifespan of intact (•) and unilaterally ovariectomized (o) CFLP mice. Animals with intact ovaries produced 96 live young *in toto* by 271 days of age (mean age at final parturition), whereas those having only one ovary from early adulthood delivered 48 young by 226 days. The opportunity for reproduction was maximized in both groups by the continuous presence of fertile males and the removal of pups at birth. (From Gosden, 1979.)

that fewer blastocysts survived after transfer from young donor mice to parous horns of unilaterally ovariectomized animals rather than to intact controls (Gosden, 1979). There may be other reasons besides uterine ageing for the early loss of fertility, such as the increasing incidence of aneuploid embryos which have been observed (Brook et al., 1984).

An experiment carried out by the distinguished eighteenth-century anatomist and surgeon, John Hunter (1728–1793), is pertinent to discussions of parity. He compared the long-term breeding performance of two sows from the same farrow, one of which had been unilaterally ovariectomized. This experiment was designed to distinguish two opposing hypotheses: (1) that each ovary can produce only a fixed number of ova during the lifespan, in which case extirpation of one should halve the total number of offspring; (2) that breeding performance is limited by constitutional factors, in which case ovariectomy would not have a major effect. He reported that the ovariectomized sow bred for only 4 years and produced 76 piglets, whereas the control animal continued to breed for an additional 2 years, yielding a total of 162 piglets (Fig. 5.10). Hunter concluded, ''It seems most probable that the ovaria are from the beginning destined to produce a fixed number, beyond which they cannot go, . . . but that the constitution at large has no power of giving to one ovarium the power of propagating equal to both; for in the present experiment the animal with one ovarium produced 10 pigs less than half the number brought forth by the sow with both ovaria'' (Hunter, 1787). Since litter sizes were maintained in the animal with only one ovary, his experiment provides the first evidence that ovulation rate is controlled globally (p. 45). It cannot, however, be used to support the postulated effect of fetal crowding because in this species embryos can become distributed evenly between the two horns, irrespective of their origin, whereas, in rodents, intrauterine migration is prevented by an anatomical barrier (Biggers et al., 1962). Thus, the poorer breeding performance of the ovariectomized sow may turn out to depend on ovarian (rather than uterine) ageing, vindicating Hunter's conclusion. The experiment needs repeating, but modern biologists faced with the dual problems of time and expense will find sympathy with Hunter's excuse: ''It may be thought by some that I should have repeated this experiment, but an annual expense of £20 for 10 years, and the necessary attention to make the experiment complete, will be a sufficient reason for my not having done it''.

The underlying mechanisms responsible for the detrimental effects of fetal crowding in rodents have not yet been identified, nor is it clear whether they are significant under normal conditions of breeding. Poor uterine vascular supply and extensive scarring of the uterine wall after earlier implantation are hypotheses worth testing. The infertility of elderly primigravidae might be explained by the unnatural pattern of repeated cycles of oestrogenic stimulation of the endometrium or by earlier onset of irregular cycles, which heralds the end of cyclic life. Either of these hypotheses could explain why fertility is restored to long-

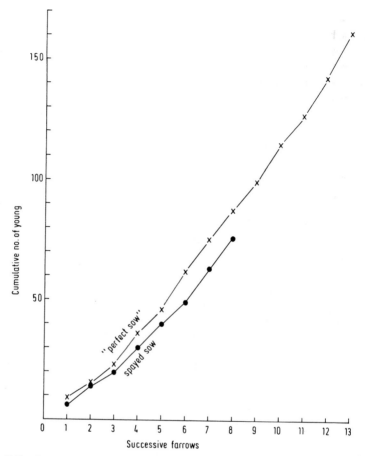

Fig. 5.10. Long-term reproductive performance of one intact ("perfect") and one unilaterally ovariectomized sow. (Adapted from Hunter, 1787.)

term castrated mice of post-reproductive age by transplanting ovaries from young donors (Felicio *et al.*, 1984).

5.4. Contraception in Middle Age

Demographic statistics clearly show that older women in many countries have successfully regulated their fertility (Table 5.1). In recent years, the fertility rates of older women have fallen dramatically, especially in Western nations. For example, the live birth rate among Scottish mothers aged 40 and over fell by

79.9% between 1950 and 1980, whereas national fertility fell by only 8.6%. Undoubtedly, many social and economic factors have contributed to this shift. In addition, there is greater public awareness of the mortality and morbidity associated with late pregnancy, although the risks for healthy women enjoying good obstetric care have sometimes been exaggerated.

The natural fertility of women wanes from the third decade of life, but a residual capacity for pregnancy remains in some individuals until menopause. Therefore, precautions against pregnancy are required in middle age, and it is prudent to maintain them for at least 1–2 years after the last natural menses. Many couples who have completed their desired family choose sterilization of one partner, but other couples prefer the reversibility of contraception, in which case the method will be dictated by personal circumstances such as medical history, frequency of coitus and attitudes to unplanned pregnancy. Reliability is often an uppermost consideration when choosing contraceptives, and it is worth pointing out that a substantial margin of safety can be gained by combining the efficiency of a contraceptive with the decreased natural fertility of ageing. For example, if a contraceptive of only 90% efficiency in young fertile groups is combined with a loss of fertility of 90%, then according to a general probability model (Biggers, 1976), the overall degree of protection is $100 [1 - (1 - 0.90)^2] =$ 99%, assuming that they act independently. This consideration should, in theory, make the simple but less reliable methods of contraception more attractive for older couples, particularly where the more sophisticated ones carry an increased risk of disease. However, it has not been possible to quantify the natural loss of fertility for individuals. Clearly, there is a need for new contraceptives which can be prescribed safely and continuously for 2 or 3 decades until middle age, but for the present, we can only discuss the suitability of the familiar methods.

Hormonal Methods

Hormonal methods include some of the most effective reversible methods of contraception and are now employed by millions of women worldwide. However, clinical research and epidemiological surveys have shown that prolonged steroid contraception may increase the risk of a number of serious diseases, e.g. myocardial infarction, thromboembolism, liver and gallbladder disease and cancer of the cervix and breast (Royal College of General Practitioners' Oral Contraception Study, 1977; Vessey *et al.*, 1977, 1983; Jick *et al.*, 1978a; Pike *et al.*, 1983). Although the evidence for some of these diseases is not as well established as for others, the International Planned Parenthood Federation, the U.S. Food and Drug Administration and other authoritative bodies have advised women over 40 years of age to choose alternative methods of contraception. Some authorities recommend an upper limit for oral contraceptive use of 35 or even 30 years, whereas others take a more circumspect view and emphasize the overriding importance of predisposing factors, such as smoking and medical history (Greenblatt *et al.*, 1979). It is unlikely that early agreement will emerge concerning the absolute levels of risk incurred by prolonged steroid contraception because the technical difficulties of obtaining reliable and representative data are now compounded by the shift in recent years to lower-dose preparations (<50 µg ethinyl oestradiol or mestranol). The possible hazards of using preparations containing oestrogen are unlikely to be overcome by switching to ones containing only progestogen because, although the side effects on metabolism are minor (Howard *et al.*, 1982), these contraceptives carry the important disadvantage of occasional breakthrough bleeding. All irregular bleeding in older women requires investigation because of the possibility of pelvic disorders, including malignant disease.

Intra-Uterine Devices

Intra-uterine devices (IUDs) are suitable for parous women who are free of menorrhagia, fibromyomata and anatomical deformations of the uterus or cervix.

Barrier Methods

Diaphragms, spermicidal jellies and condoms can be highly effective when used properly, and some carry the additional benefit of protection from sexually transmitted diseases. Such methods may be appropriate for older couples, especially where steroids or IUDs are contraindicated, but diaphragms and condoms cannot be worn on organs which have lost their tone, and the latter might exacerbate any loss of male potency.

Coitus Interruptus

Coitus interruptus, perhaps the most ancient method of birth control, is still widely practised despite its unreliability and tendency to reduce satisfaction.

Rhythm Methods

Rhythm methods depend on abstinence from coitus at the fertile time of the cycle, which is identified from calendar records of menstruation or analysis of basal body temperature rhythms or cervical mucus. Unless cycles are regular, these methods are not recommended, and during the climacteric women should be firmly discouraged from using them.

Induced Abortion

Although not strictly a contraceptive method, abortion is frequently used as a backup when contraception fails. The number of abortions among women aged 45–49 in England and Wales in 1980 almost equalled the number of live births for the same group (525 compared to 625), and the abortion rate was about 10 times that of women aged 25–29 years. Such statistics serve to highlight current attitudes and problems associated with late fertility.

6

Somatic, Metabolic and Behavioural Consequences of Menopause

6.1. Atrophy of Epithelia

Menopause, whether spontaneous or iatrogenic, is expected to lead to atrophy of epithelia which are target tissues of oestrogen and require hormonal stimulation for normal growth and differentiation. However, the distinctions between atrophy arising from hormone withdrawal, which is reversible, and that from continuous ageing processes, which is irreversible, are sometimes difficult to find. The most clear-cut examples of oestrogen-dependent atrophy are found in the postmenopausal genital tract, in which the appearance of epithelia is a faithful, if imprecise, index of hormone concentrations.

Vagina

After withdrawal of oestrogen at menopause, atrophic changes in the vagina lead gradually to shortening of the organ and reduced compliance to applied force, perhaps because of fragmentation of elastic fibres (Lang and Aponte, 1967). Epithelial and stromal cell volumes decrease as autolytic processes predominate, and the rugae characteristic of younger ages disappear. The thickness of the stratified epithelium is reduced from 8 to 10 cell layers before menopause to as few as 3 or 4 layers afterwards (Hafez, 1982). A thin-walled vagina is vulnerable to mechanical injury and readily bleeds. This condition is aggravated by dryness caused by an impaired transudate response to erotic stimuli and may cause pain at coitus (dyspareunia). The poor response might be secondary to lower vaginal blood flow after withdrawal of oestrogen (Semmens and Wagner, 1982). However, the atrophic vagina retains an ability to respond to oestrogen without leading to hyperplasia, and in women receiving exogenous oestrogen for senile vaginitis or those producing large amounts at extra-glandular sites, the epithelium is relatively thick and well differentiated with cornified superficial cells.

Significant changes of the vaginal flora occur after menopause because the

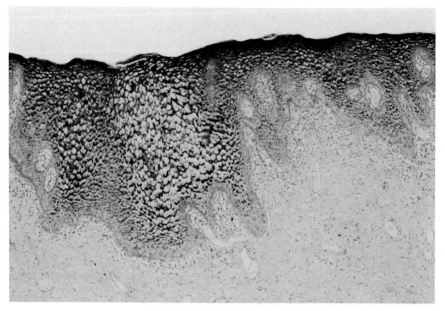

Fig. 6.1.   Vaginal epithelium of a premenopausal woman. Periodic acid-Schiff reaction (X50).

amount of glycogen associated with thinner epithelia is diminished (compare Figs. 6.1 and 6.2). Glycogen liberated from moribund and exfoliated epithelial cells provides energy for the most abundant commensals, lactobacilli (Döderleins). Since lactic acid is the end product of their metabolism, the vaginal pH is 3.5–4.5 and moderately bacteriocidal, but after menopause the pH rises above 5 (Semmens and Wagner, 1982) and the microbial population often includes staphylococci and streptococci. Thus, lower oestrogenic stimulation of the vagina is associated with a higher risk of bacterial infections; nevertheless, postmenopausal vaginitis is mainly due to yeast infections, and antibiotics may encourage their growth and make matters worse (Ross, 1978).

Urethra and Urinary Bladder

Atrophic cystitis and urethritis, loss of tone of the urinary bladder and urinary incontinence occur in many women of postmenopausal age. The lower urinary tract is sensitive to the same hormonal changes as the vagina (Smith, 1972), and both structures have stratified squamous epithelia derived from the urogenital sinus of the embryo. It is not therefore surprising that they show parallel responses to oestrogen withdrawal and treatment.

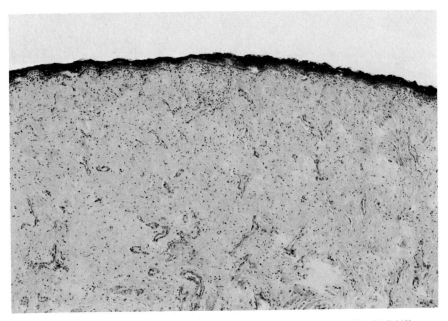

Fig. 6.2. Atrophic vaginal epithelium of a postmenopausal woman. Periodic acid-Schiff reaction (X50).

Uterus and Cervix

The overall size and cytological appearance of the uterus and cervix are strongly influenced by the amount of circulating oestrogen. The postmenopausal uterus is slowly reduced in bulk, largely because of reduced muscle, until it is a small, wedge-shaped structure less than one-quarter the dimensions of the functioning organ. The vaginal portion of the cervix may disappear altogether. The postmenopausal endometrium is typically atrophic, with a flattened, non-proliferating epithelium and glands lined by only a single layer of cells (Fig. 6.3). Glands show no cyclical changes of activity and little sign of secretion, with comparable changes occurring in the cervix uteri.

In the absence of progesterone, oestrogen of endogenous or exogenous origin can stimulate atrophic endometrial glands to proliferate, which, if prolonged, can lead to cystic changes characterized by a "Swiss cheese" appearance (Fig. 6.4). At the same time, there is hypertrophy of stromal and epithelial cells, with increased density of microvilli and cilia and the reappearance of endometrial and cervical secretions. Glandular hyperplasia is also seen in some perimenopausal women having prolonged cycles and at middle age in anovulatory rodents pre-

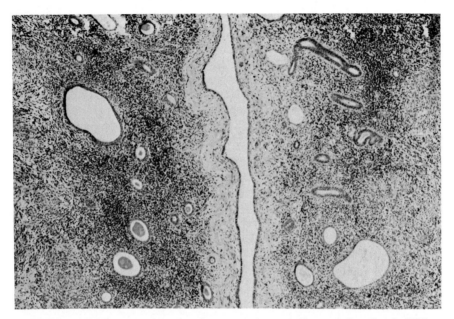

Fig. 6.3. Atrophic endometrium of a postmenopausal woman. Haematoxylin and eosin (X50).

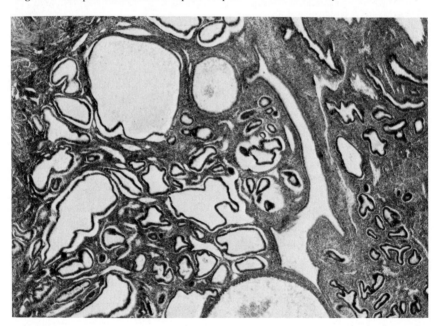

Fig. 6.4. Cystic glandular hyperplasia of the endometrium in a perimenopausal woman. Haematoxylin and eosin (X35).

senting persistent vaginal cornification. When maintained in breeding condition, virgin rabbits remain in persistent oestrus throughout most of their adult life. Chronic oestrogenic stimulation of the uterus without a luteal phase leads to hyperplasia and, hence, to adenomas and adenocarcinomas, which afflict the majority of animals at 5–6 years of age (Adams, 1970). It is a matter of concern that continuous exposure to oestrogen may cause or encourage similar diseases of the human endometrium.

Oviduct

The reduction in the length and thickness of the oviduct progresses slowly during the postmenopausal phase or following castration, but this condition can be ameliorated by administering oestrogen (Rumery and Eddy, 1974; Gaddum-Rosse et al., 1975). Smooth muscle becomes replaced by fibrous tissue, and mucosal rugae and cilia gradually disappear (Gaddum-Rosse et al., 1975; Hafez, 1982). Shortly after menopause the epithelium resembles that of cyclic women during the menstrual phase when plasma oestrogen levels reach their nadir, but after 20–30 years postmenopause substantial atrophy of ciliated and secretory cells will have taken place.

Skin

Skin is a target tissue for sex steroids. The most obvious signs of this are the sexually dimorphic plumage of birds, sex skin of primates and facial hair of men, but other widespread, if less obvious, signs are present. Human skin possesses specific cytosolic oestrogen receptors of high affinity and low capacity, but these are not uniformly distributed on the surfaces of the body (Hasselquist et al., 1980). It also contains 17α-hydroxylase, which catalyses oxidation of oestradiol to oestrone (Weinstein et al., 1968). The effects of ageing and low oestrogen status are more difficult to distinguish in skin than in the genital tract. There is no clear demonstration that exogenous oestrogens have a beneficial (i.e. cosmetic) effect on wrinkled facial skin or sagging breasts. The epidermis and dermis become thinner with increasing age after early adulthood in women and men (Punnonen, 1972; Marks and Shahrad, 1976). They lose water and elasticity and become more pigmented, and such changes are accelerated in skins regularly exposed to the ultraviolet rays in sunlight. Oestrogen seems to affect several parameters of ageing in skin, but the physiological significance of most observations is questionable because large doses have been used. In a study of ovariectomized mice, oestrone stimulated epidermal growth initially, but when administration continued, the effects were reversed and the rate of hair growth fell (Bullough, 1947). In ovariectomized women, large doses of conjugated oestrogen were found to stimulate epidermal growth but did not have the self-limiting effect observed in mice (Punnonen, 1972). Besides the effects on cell numbers, oestrogen stimulated the synthesis, maturation and turnover of collagen in animals, but the net result of prolonged treatment was to decrease amounts overall (Smith and Allison, 1966; Henneman, 1968). After castration, animals deposit more fat in their subcutaneous tissues and deep body sites, and it is probable that human menopause is one factor which predisposes middle-aged women to obesity.

The skin of the vulva shows conspicuous changes after middle age which are independent of oestrogen levels. It becomes delicate and parchment-like, and may show hyperplastic and hyperkeratotic alternation (''kraurosis vulvae'') (Lang and Aponte, 1967). Wrinkling occurs through loss of subcutaneous fat, and hair follicles become sparse. Hair is lost at many sites of the body, but at a few sites it grows more thickly (e.g. the chin and upper lip), which has been attributed to a higher androgen : oestrogen ratio after menopause.

6.2. Autonomic Nervous Disturbances

The major vasomotor disorders of the climacteric are hot flushes (flashes), palpitations and headaches. The first is probably the most common climacteric symptom, affecting three out of four women to some degree. Flushing episodes begin shortly before or after the last menses and persist for a few years, but there is considerable individual variation, and in exceptional cases these episodes continue for 20 or more years (Table 1.1). Their frequency varies from several each day to one or two per week.

The symptoms are well defined. There is a prodromal phase in which women describe sensations of pressure in the head (rather like a headache) which increase in intensity, and the flush is felt within the following 4 min. The flush itself is characterized by a feeling of heat commencing in the head and neck which then passes to the shoulders and chest region. Physiological recordings show cutaneous vasodilatation with sweating in most regions of the body, but subjects are not always aware how widespread these effects are. These symptoms are distressing, especially in social contexts, and are sometimes responsible for insomnia, which may benefit from oestrogen treatment of flushing (Kupperman et al., 1959; Hagen et al., 1982a). Similar symptoms commence within a few days of bilateral ovariectomy in women of premenopausal age (Aksel et al., 1976).

Physiological studies have countered earlier claims that hot flushes are entirely psychosomatic. It is surprising how few measurements have been made in view of the number of women affected and the interesting biological nature of the phenomenon. Molnar (1975) was the first to carry out physiological measurements of hot flushes, but he studied only one subject. Most observers agree that

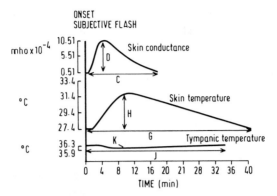

ONSET
SUBJECTIVE FLASH

Fig. 6.5. Changes in skin conductance, skin temperature and core temperature (tympanic membrane) associated with 25 hot flushes in climacteric women. Mean values are shown. (From Tataryn *et al.*, 1980; reprinted with permission.)

the first objective sign of a flushing episode is a rise in skin conductance (a function of the rate of sweating) beginning about 45 sec after the subjective premonition (Sturdee *et al.*, 1978; Tataryn *et al.*, 1980). Conductance is maximal about 4 min later and declines to baseline in a further 14 min (Fig. 6.5). The concomitant rise of skin temperature is of longer duration and is more variable in extent, being highest in the toes and fingers (c. 4°C), perhaps because of less cooling by evaporation of sweat. Skin temperature changes are generally less reliable as indicators of the time course of the flushing episode than changes in conductance (Tataryn *et al.*, 1980).

During climacteric flushing the rate of blood flowing to the hand rises three–fourfold in the first 2–3 min and is maintained at the higher level for a few minutes longer before returning rapidly to baseline (Fig. 6.6). The time course of similar changes in forearm and finger blood flows are slightly different. Since skeletal muscle and skin each receive their distinctive types of vasomotor innervation, it is probable that these haemodynamic changes are confined to cutaneous vessels. The flush is accompanied by a rising heart rate of 20% over resting values, but there are no changes in blood pressure or circulating catecholamines or irregularities of the electrocardiogram (Sturdee *et al.*, 1978; Casper *et al.*, 1979; Ginsburg *et al.*, 1981). The sweating and peripheral vasodilatation lead to an increased heat loss by evaporation and radiation and, hence, to a fall in core body temperature by about 0.2°C (Fig. 6.5).

Since flushing and sweating are associated with ovarian failure and are usually alleviated by exogenous oestrogens, they have been assumed to be consequences of oestrogen deficiency, either directly or indirectly. In some studies, symptomatic women had lower levels of oestradiol and/or oestrone than asymptomatic individuals at perimenopausal ages (Campbell, 1976; Chakravarti *et al.*, 1979;

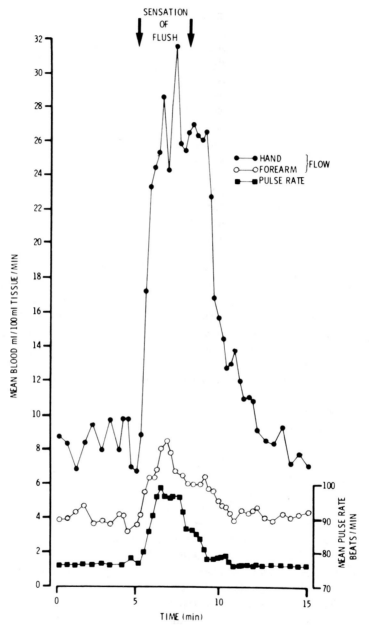

Fig. 6.6. Mean hand and forearm blood flow and pulse rate in six women before, during and after a perimenopausal hot flush. (From Ginsburg *et al.*, 1981; reprinted with permission.)

Hagen *et al.*, 1982b), but in other studies no distinction was seen (Aksel *et al.*, 1976; Chakravarti *et al.*, 1977; Badawy *et al.*, 1979). The vasomotor disorders can be attributed to habituation of neurons to oestrogen after puberty. When hormone levels fall profoundly in mid-life a period of metabolic adjustment to the new internal environment is required. If there is a critical period for habituation it must be brief because teenage girls have reported flushing after ovarian failure or castration. These observations seem to be at variance with findings from hypogonadal women with Turner's syndrome, in whom symptoms are totally lacking despite the fact that 30% of them experience some menstrual activity and many receive exogenous oestrogens (W. H. Price, personal communication).

There are strong indications that climacteric flushing is neither a direct nor a specific effect of oestrogen withdrawal. Flushing has been recorded after hypothalamic damage in a small number of girls and boys at early stages of puberty, i.e. without exposure to adult female levels of oestrogens (Witt and Blethen, 1983). In double-blind trials, adult symptoms have been alleviated significantly by treatment with placebos and progestogens, and the benefits of the latter have sometimes approached those obtained with oestrogens (Dennerstein *et al.*, 1978; Paterson, 1982; Lobo *et al.*, 1984). Also, non-hormonal substances such as clonidine and naloxone have been reported to be effective (Clayden *et al.*, 1974; Lightman *et al.*, 1981), but negative results have been obtained more recently (Lindsay and Hart, 1978; DeFazio *et al.*, 1984). Flushing is frequently experienced by hypogonadal men soon after castration or treatment with LHRH agonists, the peripheral physiological changes being similar to those of climacteric women (Ginsburg and O'Reilly, 1983). These observations imply that withdrawal of androgens or possibly other non-oestrogenic gonadal secretions can trigger vasomotor disorders.

Although pituitary gonadotrophins rise during the climacteric, they cannot be held responsible for these symptoms. Neither exogenous gonadotrophins nor LHRH trigger symptoms in young women. Moreover, hot flushes and sweating occur after hypophysectomy when levels of gonadotrophins are lowered (Mulley *et al.*, 1977; Meldrum *et al.*, 1981b). A notable synchrony between flushing episodes, identified by rising finger temperature, and pulsatile release of LH has been found (Tataryn *et al.*, 1979; Casper *et al.*, 1979). Because FSH pulses are less clearly defined, it is not certain whether these are also synchronized (Fig. 6.7). No such relationship has been found with oestrogen levels, although plasma dehydroepiandrosterone levels are elevated during flushing and may be secondary to stressful effects of symptoms (Meldrum *et al.*, 1980). That the pulses of LH are not responsible for flushes has been demonstrated by two types of experiments, each using superactive LHRH analogues to inhibit pulsatile release of LH by down-regulating pituitary LHRH receptors. The analogues produced flushing in premenopausal women by lowering gonadotrophins and, hence, go-

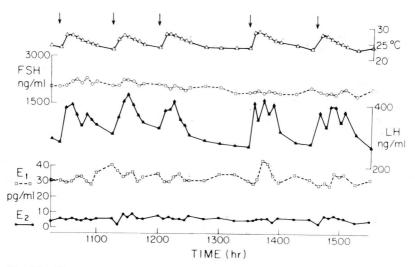

Fig. 6.7. Simultaneous measurements in a climacteric woman of hot flushes (onset marked by arrows which indicate increased finger temperature), serum FSH, LH, oestrone (E_1) and oestradiol (E_2). (From Meldrum *et al.*, 1980; reprinted with permission.)

nadal secretion (DeFazio *et al.*, 1983) and were unable to relieve spontaneous symptoms in climacteric women (Casper and Yen, 1981).

Since each pulse of LH corresponds to a pulse of LHRH neurosecretion (Clarke and Cummins, 1982), flushing symptoms would seem to have a central origin. This hypothesis is strengthened by the following points: (1) Objective signs of flushing are often preceded by premonitions. (2) There is the theoretical difficulty of explaining how vasodilatation, involving adrenergic fibres, and sweat gland excitation, involving sympathetic cholinergic fibres, could both be triggered by a common peripheral factor carried in the circulation. On the other hand, this dual activity is wholly consistent with the physiological property of increasing sympathetic drive centrally under circumstances that require the core temperature to be lowered. (3) The fall in core temperature during the flush is itself an indication of a central disorder since peripheral cooling would be expected to lead to thermoregulatory adjustments to abrogate any fall in core temperature (Judd and Korenman, 1982). There is therefore good reason to believe that vasomotor symptoms are the result of inappropriate activity of central thermoregulatory mechanisms (Tataryn *et al.*, 1980).

Central thermoreceptors are located in the posterior preoptic–anterior hypothalamic areas, not far from the hypothalamic LHRH-containing neurons which are influenced during flushing. The initiating event of the hot flush seems to cause a transient fall of the set point of the central thermostat. A set point in a regulatory system is that value of a controlled variable at which control action is zero. A fall therefore indicates the need to dissipate heat and brings about peripheral changes leading to lower core temperature.

The cellular mechanism by which withdrawal of oestrogen affects the central thermoregulatory set point is not known. One possibility which is currently under study is that decreasing levels of catechol oestrogen, which correspond to the postmenopausal withdrawal of classical oestrogens, lead to thermoregulatory instability by affecting monoaminergic synapses. The catechol oestrogens, which are products of metabolizing oestradiol and oestrone (see Section 2.4), are cleared so rapidly from blood that circulating amounts are unlikely to be high enough to have physiological effects (Merriam *et al.*, 1980), but those formed in the hypothalamus might be sufficient to exert a localized influence on neurones (Fishman and Norton, 1975). Because of their structural similarity, the 2-hydroxyoestrogens are potent competitive inhibitors of the metabolism of catecholamines by catechol-*o*-methyltransferase (Ball *et al.*, 1972; Lloyd *et al.*, 1978). On the other hand, they displace catecholamines from cellular binding sites, at least in non-neural tissue (Schaeffer and Hsueh, 1979), and affect catecholamine synthesis by inhibiting the rate-limiting enzyme, tyrosine hydroxylase (Lloyd and Weisz, 1978). The net effect of these opposing actions of catechol oestrogens on synaptic activity is not predictable, though the findings provide grounds for suspecting their involvement in climacteric flushing.

6.3. Demineralization of Bone

Demineralization of bone is potentially the most serious long-term consequence of human menopause. Not only does it cause immense suffering to individuals, but it is also costly to the community. Excessive loss of bone leads to clinical osteoporosis, which is responsible for an increasing incidence of bone fractures among older women (Nordin *et al.*, 1980a). All parts of the axial and appendicular skeleton become progressively rarefied after menopause, but it is the distal forearm, neck of the femur and spine that have the greatest risk of fracture. Spinal fractures are diagnostic of osteoporosis in old age because they occur spontaneously when there is insufficient trabecular bone to act as supporting cross braces, leading to compression damage (Twomey *et al.*, 1983). Limb bones are fractured by traumatic accident, the femoral neck being the most important site because it is a significant cause of death in elderly women. The incidence of this fracture rises exponentially after age 50; by the ninth decade the cumulative incidence in an American population was 32% in women but only 17% in men (Gallagher *et al.*, 1980a). Thus, there is good reason for the current attention on the pathophysiology of bone loss in postmenopause.

Albright *et al.* (1941) were first to recognize a higher frequency of osteoporotic patients amongst postmenopausal women, but the importance of their discovery was insufficiently appreciated at the time. Meema (1966) and Nordin *et al.* (1966) showed that commencement of bone loss depended on postmenopausal status rather than chronological age, and it soon became apparent that this is not due to the presence of diseases which are recognised causes of bone deterioration, viz. renal failure, hyperparathyroidism, thyrotoxicosis and Cushing's syndrome. On the basis of the epidemiology of osteoporosis and the pattern of cortical and trabecular bone loss, two distinct syndromes of differing aetiology have been identified. Type I osteoporosis is associated with oestrogen deficiency after the menopause. Type II ("senile osteoporosis") afflicts a proportion of much older women (>75 years) and involves accelerated bone loss with poor absorption of calcium (Riggs and Melton, 1983). Unfortunately, this distinction has not always been made, which could explain some conflicting data.

Several methods for measuring bone mass are available. X-ray film densitometry and γ-ray and X-ray absorptiometry are commonly used for measuring cortical bone thickness of the appendages, the second metacarpal of the right hand being the site favoured by many research groups. Trabecular bone can be assessed simply by an X-ray film of the proximal femur, but for quantitative information biopsies of the iliac crest are taken for histomorphometry. Progressive changes in bone density can be monitored readily in longitudinal studies of individual women. In cross-sectional studies, values obtained with these methods must be corrected for total bone volume because osteoporosis is defined according to the relative amounts of bone lost (mass : volume ratio); otherwise all women with small bones would be assigned to this category.

These methods have provided unequivocal evidence that both cortical and trabecular bone are lost in postmenopausal women. During the early postmenopausal phase, the rate of trabecular bone loss is the greater of the two, but because this component represents only 20% of the skeleton at most, the rate falls after age 60 because of the limited amounts remaining (Crilly *et al.*, 1981). Hence, the incidence of spinal fractures does not rise continuously in old age, in contrast to that of hip fractures, which depend on loss of both cortical and trabecular bone. The rate of cortical bone loss is greater during the first 3 years of postmenopause than afterwards (−2.7% compared to −0.7% annually in the study of Lindsay *et al.*, 1976), which, in a general way, parallels the slow metabolic adjustment of the thermoregulatory apparatus to lower levels of oestrogen. The rates of bone loss might seem small, but since losses are cumulative, they are highly significant in the long run. Bone is also lost in ageing men, though a later onset and a lower rate of loss afford them greater protection against fractures in old age (Dequecker *et al.*, 1971).

Since 99% of body calcium is located in the skeleton and all bones tend to become porous in advancing years, measurements of total body calcium (TbCa) using neutron activation analysis provide a valuable guide to global changes of bone density. In this method a beam of partially moderated, fast neutrons from a cyclotron or other source is directed towards the subject, in whom the reaction $^{48}Ca(n,\gamma)^{49}Ca$ is induced, besides other elemental changes (Cohn, 1980). The dose of radiation absorbed is small (c. 0.3 rem) and can therefore be repeated for longitudinal studies. Radioisotopes generated in tissue emit a spectrum of γ radiation which is specific for each element and can be detected in a whole body counter. Such methods are readily standardized and are less dependent on subjective criteria than those mentioned above. The TbCa of normal, healthy white Americans is shown in Fig. 6.8. Individual values are highly variable; nevertheless, two findings are outstanding: (1) Those of women are 20–40% lower than those of men of the same age, reflecting differences in body size. (2) The TbCa declines from middle age in women, but this decline is less marked in men. Cohn *et al.* (1976) divided the data for women into two sets by imposing an arbitrary age of 55 to separate pre- and postmenopausal groups. The rate of loss of TbCa was estimated to be 0.38% annually in those aged 35–54, rising to

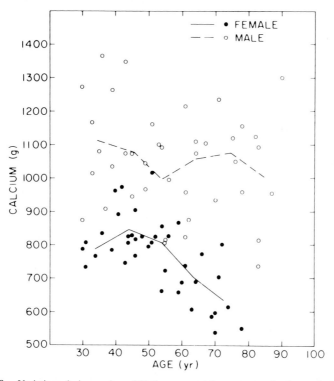

Fig. 6.8. Variations during ageing of TbCa measured by neutron activation analysis. Curves were drawn from mean values for each decade for women and men. (From Cohn *et al.*, 1976; reprinted with permission.)

1.08% in women aged 55–79. These figures imply that 95 mmoles (3.8 g) and 190 mmoles (7.6 g) of calcium are lost annually in pre- and postmenopausal women, respectively. Thus, by age 79, 6.25 moles (250 g) of calcium will have been lost, which amounts to about 28% of the TbCa of women aged 30. The amounts of phosphorus lost during life are in close accord with theoretical predictions based on the stoichiometric relationship to calcium. These important data are marred only by the assumption of the late menopausal age of 55. The rate of bone loss in young women may, therefore, have been seriously overestimated by combining a low (if existent) premenopausal value with higher values in postmenopausal women. Such doubts have been strengthened by Kennedy *et al.* (1982), who found that the TbCa was stable in premenopausal women but subsequently declined at an annual rate of 1.5%. Neither study was able to verify whether postmenopausal bone loss commences at a high rate and falls later; longitudinal studies of individual women will be required to test this hypothesis. The extent to which ageing men become demineralized also requires further study. Cohn *et al.* (1976) estimated the annual rate of loss of calcium was 0.7%, whereas Kennedy *et al.* (1982) were unable to find any significant change during ageing.

There are surprisingly large ethnic and national differences in the age-specific incidence of bone fractures. Anecdotal evidence suggests that old women in some parts of the developing world are less vulnerable to fractures than those elsewhere (World Health Organization, 1981). There is little doubt that in this regard older American black women have a strong advantage over American whites (Iskrant, 1968). The greater total body levels of calcium and phosphorus in these black women at most ages, even after adjusting for differences in height and weight, would appear to explain these differences (Cohn *et al.*, 1977). Progressive demineralization during ageing might be a general phenomenon, but whether it leads to fragile bones will depend on life expectancy after menopause, mineralization in early adulthood, diet and other factors.

Albright *et al.* (1941) assumed that postmenopausal osteoporosis is caused by diminished formation of new bone, but this has turned out to be incorrect. Most evidence indicates that bone remodelling is increased during ageing, the rate of resorption exceeding that of new bone formation (Riggs *et al.*, 1969; Heaney *et al.*, 1978b; Delmas *et al.*, 1983). After menopause, fasting levels of urinary hydroxyproline and plasma alkaline phosphatase rise, these being non-specific indicators of bone resorption (Crilly *et al.*, 1981). The process of resorption is responsible for higher plasma levels of calcium and phosphate in fasting postmenopausal and castrated women (Young and Nordin, 1967; Gallagher *et al.*, 1972), but these levels rarely exceed the upper limit of the normal range and do not therefore lead to clinical hypercalcaemia. The effects of ageing and menopause on phosphate excretion are more controversial and depend on the circulating amounts of parathyroid hormone, which are affected, in turn, by blood calcium levels (see below). Many of the changes associated with postmenopausal bone loss are small, subtle deviations within the normal physiological range. If considered singly these changes might be overlooked, but they are significant over long periods of time.

Many clinical studies have shown that exogenous oestrogens inhibit bone loss in postmenopausal women (World Health Organization, 1981). This treatment can even lead to a net increase in bone material if sufficiently large doses are given (>25μg ethinyl oestradiol/day) (Christiansen *et al.*, 1982; Horsman *et al.*, 1983). Most oestrogens can prevent bone loss, but oestriol requires continuous administration in large doses (Lindsay *et al.*, 1979). Conservation of bone reduces the risk of fractures later in life. In an American study, the risks of fracturing either the distal forearm or the hip were reduced 50–60% when oestrogen treatment had continued for at least 6 years (Weiss *et al.*, 1980). To be fully effective, treatment should commence at menopause and continue indefinitely. In one study, withdrawal of treatment led to a high rate of bone loss which cancelled out benefits accruing from earlier conservation (Lindsay *et al.*, 1978), but some other studies have shown that long-term protection is afforded even by limited treatment with oestrogens (Christiansen *et al.*, 1981).

The prophylactic effects of exogenous oestrogens suggest, but do not prove, that the loss of bone mineral content in postmenopausal women is due to a deficiency of follicular oestrogen. Some studies show plasma oestrogen levels are related inversely to fasting urinary levels of calcium, hydroxyproline and the degree of metacarpal bone loss; these elements being of a more physiological nature, provide firmer support of the hypothesis (Frumar *et al.*, 1980; Crilly *et al.*, 1981). However, a relationship between oestrogen levels and clinical osteoporosis has not been established. Marshall *et al.* (1977) found osteoporotic women had lower circulating levels of oestrone than age-matched controls. Davidson *et al.* (1982, 1983) were unable to confirm this result in patients with hip fractures, although sex steroid-binding globulin activity was raised. A higher incidence of postmenopausal osteoporosis among non-obese than obese women (Daniell, 1976; Davidson *et al.*, 1982) might be accounted for by lower production of oestrogen and/or less biologically active circulating oestrogen (see Section 2.3). If women require oestrogen to maintain bone mineral content at young adult levels, young hypogonadal women would be expected to be particularly vulnerable to fractures and so would be expected to require hormonal therapy throughout life. But, paradoxically, women with Turner's syndrome do not become rapidly demineralized, nor do they have a high risk of fractures late in life (Smith *et al.*, 1982). Presumably, they are either protected by a special feature of their constitution or they have not been exposed to sufficient oestrogen for a withdrawal response to occur.

Many explanations have been offered for the protective effects of oestrogen on bone mineral status in postmenopausal women. The effects may turn out to be indirect for, despite a thorough search, high-affinity cytosolic receptors for oestrogen have not been detected in bone (Chen and Feldman, 1978; van Paassen *et al.*,1978). The significance, if any, of aromatase activity in this tissue is therefore obsure (Vittek *et al.*, 1974; Frisch *et al.*, 1980). Consequently, more attention is now being focussed on possible mediating effects of other hormones involved in calcium homeostasis.

The thyroid hormone, calcitonin, has been considered as a possible mediator of the protective effects of oestrogen on bone minerals. Calcitonin conserves bone calcium and opposes the resorptive activities of parathyroid hormone and vitamin D. The suspicion that calcitonin is deficient after menopause is rein-forced by circumstantial evidence that plasma levels are lower in women than in men and are increased by exogenous oestrogen (Morimoto *et al.*, 1980; Steven-son *et al.*, 1981). Moreover, ovariectomy in rats impairs the normal release of calcitonin by calcium salts, this effect being reversed by oestrogen treatment (Catherwood *et al.*, 1983). In women this response to calcium wanes slowly throughout adult life without an abrupt change at menopausal age, and so oestrogen withdrawal is not likely to be a prime cause of lower calcitonin (Shamonki *et al.*, 1980). Conflicting results have been obtained when blood calcitonin levels were analysed in osteoporotic women. In one study levels were sub-normal (Milhaud *et al.*, 1978), but in another study they were not related to the severity of the disease (Chestnut *et al.*, 1980). Firm conclusions cannot be drawn at this stage, but it is unlikely that insufficient calcitonin is entirely responsible for demineralization after menopause.

Parathyroid hormone has also been considered to be a potential agent of postmenopausal bone loss because it is a hypercalcaemic hormone which can withdraw mineral stored in the skeleton, besides promoting calcium retention by acting on the kidneys and gut. Organ culture studies have shown that oestrogen inhibits the ability of parathyroid hormone to release calcium and phosphate from mouse calvaria (Atkins *et al.*, 1972), but the interpretation of these data is made difficult by the studies which failed to find cytosolic receptors in other bones. The circulating levels of parathyroid hormone have been found to be slightly elevated during normal ageing as well as in osteoporotic patients (Insogna *et al.*, 1981; Delmas *et al.*, 1983; Marcus *et al.*, 1984). These levels could be a physiological response to poor absorption of calcium. Oestrogen might affect the actions of other hormones, leading to a negative calcium balance, e.g. by affect-ing actions of growth hormone (Schwartz *et al.*, 1969), or by some undefined mechanism leading to greater catabolism of the collagenous matrix of bone (Smith and Allison, 1966; Henneman, 1968).

Bone mineral loss is aggravated by an inadequate intake of calcium, which may partly explain why the rates of loss are so variable between individuals. Calcium deficiency is attributed to a poor diet (low calcium content and/or bound to phytate) or an impaired ability of the gut to absorb available calcium, a condition which is prevalent among ageing women, especially those with severe osteoporosis (Ireland and Fordtran, 1973; Gallagher *et al.*, 1979; Crilly *et al.*, 1981). Poor absorption could arise from vitamin D deficiency because vitamin levels are often marginal or inadequate in elderly women, especially during the winter months at higher latitudes. However, this should not imply that histological features of osteoporosis and osteomalacia are necessarily concurrent; indeed, in an English study the histological features of these distinct conditions were combined in only 10% of cases (Nordin *et al.*, 1980a). Small doses of vitamin D improved the absorption of calcium in short-term studies of osteoporotic women (Gallagher *et al.*, 1982), but primary failure of the absorptive mechanism in the small intestine was important in some cases (Francis *et al.*, 1984). Oestrogen may help to preserve the status of vitamin D by directly or indirectly stimulating renal 1α-hydroxylase activity to bring about formation of the active metabolite, 1,25-dihydroxycholecalciferol. Of these two alternatives, the indirect pathway is more probable, namely, that oestrogen inhibits the transferral of calcium from bone to blood (by some elusive mechanism), allowing levels of parathyroid hormone to rise, which then acts on the kidney (Gallagher *et al.*, 1980b). Low calcium intake is an important factor contributing to demineralization of the skeleton, but the greater urinary excretion of calcium indicates that its role is secondary.

To sum up, it has not been possible to demonstrate a simple causal nexus between lower oestrogen levels and demineralization after menopause. Nevertheless, oestrogen is suspected of having some kind of protective effect on bones of normal women. Human biologists will have to surmount many technical problems, as well as uncover interactive factors in clarifying the causes of osteoporosis. Besides the widespread and complex metabolic changes after menopause, there are continuously changing patterns of life-style which could be as relevant. The significance of vitamin D status and calcium content of the diet has already been stressed, and to it must be added the detrimental effects of physical inactivity on bone condition. Further reference to these factors is made in the next chapter because small changes in life-style might have lasting benefits.

6.4. Intermediary Metabolism

The effects of oestrogen on cellular metabolism and growth and the consequences of oestrogen deficiency after menopause have been discussed in many sections of this book. But, so far, there has been no discussion of whether metabolic changes arising from oestrogen withdrawal promote major degenerative diseases of middle and old age. Loss of ovarian activity does not appear to affect the metabolism of carbohydrates in normal healthy women (Notelovitz,

1982), nor is thyroid activity altered (Baschieri *et al.*, 1982). However, serum levels of cholesterol and triglycerides rise after menopause. These changes are significant risk factors for cardiovascular disease from which women are invariably spared until postmenopause (Hjortland *et al.*, 1976; Lindquist and Bengtsson, 1980). It is probably their oestrogens that afford young women protection from disease rather than age itself, since bilateral ovariectomy leads to a precocious rise in both serum lipids and the risk of disease among individuals of premenopausal age (Oliver and Boyd, 1959; Gordon *et al.*, 1978; Rosenberg *et al.*, 1981). In addition, after menopause the proportion of cholesterol carried by high density lipoproteins falls to values similar to those found in men of all ages (Barr, 1953). These lipoproteins are responsible for transporting effete cholesterol from peripheral tissues, including arterial walls, to liver for catabolism and excretion (Miller and Miller, 1975). In epidemiological studies an inverse relationship has been found to exist between high density lipoprotein cholesterol and risk of cardiovascular disease (Gordon *et al.*, 1977), which strengthens suspicions that atherogenesis is promoted by withdrawal of oestrogen. However, the aetiology of ischaemic heart disease in postmenopausal women is likely to be more complex than this, perhaps involving rising levels of serum triglycerides (Riemersma, 1984) and of factors involved in haemostatic function leading to greater coagulability (Meade *et al.*, 1983).

6.5. Sexual Behaviour

Circulating levels of sex steroids fall after menopause, but it is doubtful whether they can fully account for the reputed decline in sexual interest and activity of ageing. Human sexual behaviour is the most complex variable mentioned so far and is affected by biological, psychological and sociological factors. Only for animals can it be stated with confidence that hypogonadism abolishes the sexual response.

Female rodents are sexually receptive for only a few hours around the time of ovulation. During this brief period of "oestrus" they adopt a "lordotic" posture (Gk. *lordosis:* bent backwards) to allow mounting and penetration by the male. Synchrony of sexual behavior and ovulation is achieved by the same internal signals, namely, exposure of the brain to gonadal steroids, especially oestrogen. Progesterone has a potentiating effect in animals primed with oestrogen, but it inhibits lordosis under other circumstances. Although details differ between species, the ovarian steroids are essential for receptivity in all higher animals, including sub-human primates (Michael and Bonsall, 1977).

In old age, when production of sex steroids falls because of a dwindling store of ovarian follicles, rodents become sexually unreceptive (anoestrus). However, most strains do not reach this phase, but instead enter one of persistent vaginal cornification, with moderately elevated levels of oestrogen remaining for much of postcyclic life (p. 71). During this anovulatory phase, multiparous rats aged 19 months old were frequently, but not uniformly, receptive to males. Coitus temporarily interrupted their acyclical vaginal smear pattern, suggesting that neuroendocrine responses had been elicited (Cooper and Linnoila, 1977; Hendricks *et al.*, 1979). Individual differences in receptivity probably depended on oestrogen levels because rats having vaginal smears containing a mixture of cornified cells and leucocytes (probably indicative of less oestrogenic stimulation) rarely allowed mounting to occur. On the other hand, when ageing animals presented short cycles their lordosis behaviour was indistinguishable from that of young animals, as was that of ovariectomized rats receiving gonadal steroid replacement treatment at ages 20–30 months (Peng *et al.*, 1977). Therefore, the brain and motor systems of old rats with breeding experience are capable of normal sexual responses given appropriate priming by hormones.

These findings should not be extrapolated to our own species because of the strong influence of non-biological factors on human sexuality. Valid comparisons cannot be made because our sexuality is generally measured as "libido", a vague subjective measure of sex drive, whereas, in rodents, a specific response (lordosis) is measured. It is still not clear to what extent physiological levels of sex steroids affect libido in women because few rigorous double-blind experiments with ovariectomized subjects have been undertaken. There is tentative evidence that a small quantity of oestrogen is required for libido, but a dose–response relationship does not exist above a low threshold (Sanders and Bancroft, 1982). Since human sexual activity is maximal at both pre- and postmenstrual stages of the cycle, oestrogen does not have such a dominating influence on behaviour as it does in animals (Bancroft, 1983). The role of other gonadal steroids in human libido is even more obscure. Testosterone has been shown to be proceptive, at least in pharmacological doses, but might require aromatization in the brain (Naftolin *et al.*, 1975). And in the case of progesterone, equivocal results have been obtained. These major uncertainties about the normal role of sex steroids inevitably limit our understanding of sexuality during ageing.

The effects of age on human sexual behaviour were studied extensively by Kinsey *et al.* (1953) in the United States. Marital coital rates at 40 years of age were half those at age 20. Sexual interest and activity in men declined continuously from puberty, whereas solitary sexual activities of unmarried women did not fall until age 55–60. The authors concluded that women do not age in their sexual capacities until late in life, and they blamed husbands for declining marital coitus. Similar conclusions were reached by James (1974b) in an English survey. Coital rates were correlated more closely with the age of the husband than with that of the wife. There was a fall by 0.8 coitions per month for every 5 additional years of the husband's age; the corresponding value for wives was only 0.1 coition when other variables were controlled. Other studies carried out in the somewhat artificial environment of the laboratory showed that postmenopausal women retained a potential for effective sexual responses, especially when regularly stimulated, although the intensity and duration at each phase were reduced (Masters and Johnson, 1966).

Some studies have found a reduction in sex drive and capacity for orgasm during the climacteric. Such findings are not necessarily in conflict with the conclusions of Kinsey *et al.* (1953) and James (1974b), who were mainly concerned with long-term changes, but they definitely refute the old notion of a flareup of sex drive in middle age (Hallström, 1979). Waning libido in climacteric women may be secondary to the physical discomfort of hot flushes, sweating and dyspareunia or to insomnia and anxiety, which are common at these ages. Sex steroid therapy might, therefore, benefit sexual pleasure indirectly by relieving these symptoms (Masters and Johnson, 1966; Morrell *et al.*, 1984).

Patterns of sexual interest and activity during and following the climacteric are highly complex and variable, and it is unwise to make sweeping conclusions. In some couples the major factors might be the attitude of the male partner or cultural restraints on sexuality, whereas in others the biological effects of menopause may be uppermost. Withdrawal of sex steroids would not appear to directly affect libido, and any benefits obtained with exogenous oestrogens are attributable to the reversal of genital atrophy and amelioration of climacteric symptoms.

7

The Hormone Replacement Therapy (HRT) Controversy

In recent years, the failure of postmenopausal human ovaries to produce oestrogen has probably been responsible for more attention on the ageing reproductive system than any other factor. This is not surprising since this failure is marked by the important landmark of menopause and is associated with unpleasant symptoms and long-term metabolic changes which extend beyond the redundancy of reproductive organs. Public interest in the subject has been heightened by the widespread use of oestrogen for "hormone replacement therapy (HRT)" in Western countries, in which a large proportion of women are of postmenopausal age. Such treatment is undoubtedly effective in alleviating those symptoms of middle age which arise from the biological effects of oestrogen withdrawal. However, the use of "replacement" hormones remains controversial because of fears of promoting serious diseases, and for individual cases the decision whether to prescribe them is not a clear-cut scientific one but requires the craft of the experienced practitioner. Nevertheless, knowledge of human biological factors forms a basis for the practical problems of management. In this concluding chapter, these factors are revisited as an introduction for readers with clinical and pharmacological interests.

First, it is necessary to consider whether postmenopause is a natural condition since the answer to this question will affect attitudes to HRT. Apart from embarking on a purely semantic argument, this question can be tackled in the following way. If "natural" implies a physiological state, the answer must be affirmative because all women reaching their seventh decade will have experienced menopause. However, the observation that menopause is universal does not lead to any fresh insight unless the phenomenon can be shown to be an evolutionary adaptation. Little evidence has been produced in support of this view. Menopause evidently is a spurious phenomenon, an inevitable consequence of lifespan extension, and a postreproductive phase of life occurs in other species under conditions which favour longevity (see Chapter 1). Apart from avoiding the higher risks associated with maternity at advanced age, individual women gain no biological advantage in postmenopause; indeed, they appear to be physiologically ill-adapted for it. The use of HRT cannot, therefore, be ruled out on the grounds that it is unnatural, but it can be justified in certain cases on pragmatic grounds.

7.1. Who Requires HRT?

It is generally agreed that HRT is not required by all women and is positively not recommended for some. Most surveys show a small proportion of women are asymptomatic during the perimenopause, though it remains to be shown whether these individuals are also relatively protected from insidious development of osteoporosis and atherosclerosis at later ages. Only weak or insignificant correlations have been found between circulating oestrogen levels and the signs and symptoms associated with menopause. Moreover, cross-cultural surveys indicate that social factors influence the appearance and intensity of climacteric symptoms (p. 6). Since the levels of oestrogen in postmenopausal women are highly variable and a sub-population of hormone-deficient individuals cannot be delineated, it is difficult to predict which women will benefit from HRT. A secondary problem is the question of whether for a given individual, treatment should be confined to symptoms during the climacteric or prolonged indefinitely for prophylaxis against osteoporosis.

Bone demineralization, which proceeds at an annual rate of about 1%, is the most serious consequence of menopause because it increases the risk of fractures, which can be fatal in the elderly woman. Exogenous oestrogen counters this tendency by inhibiting or even reversing the loss of bone substance (see Section 6.3). The risk of fractures late in life is highly variable. Caucasian women seem to be more vulnerable than those of other races, and the risk is increased for the slender and for the smoker (Daniell, 1976). A low level of oestrogen (principally oestrone) circulates in postmenopausal women, but even this may afford some protection against the loss of mineral and damage to bones. Most of this oestrogen is derived from peripheral aromatization of androstenedione of adrenal origin. Therefore, the natural tendency to lose bone is likely to be exacerbated under conditions of impaired adrenocortical function (e.g. corticosteroid therapy, adrenal disease). In contrast, the ovaries are no longer a significant source of oestrogen and only a minor source of its precursors, so their removal is unlikely to be significant. Since the extent to which the skeleton is demineralized depends on the number of years after menopause rather than on chronological age *per se,* precocious menopause, whether spontaneous or surgical, is expected to raise the risk of bone injury late in life. In addition, there is a greater possibility (though admittedly remote) of developing rare gonadotrophin-producing adenomas in the pituitary gland (Trouillas *et al.*, 1981) and, more important, coronary artery disease (p. 138). Therefore, it would seem necessary for women who have precocious menopause, but who are otherwise healthy, to begin HRT immediately after the last menses and continue medication at least until the normal age of menopause. Unfortunately, there is at present no generally agreed-upon normal age range for menopause so precocity cannot be defined by strict statistical criteria (see Section 3.7).

Another indication for HRT is for some cases of atrophy of the genito-urinary tract. These patients are likely to present with symptoms of dyspareunia and reduced interest in sexual union. Whereas these effects develop slowly and persist, vasomotor disturbances (hot flushes and sweating) tend to be confined to a few years before and after menopause. Nevertheless, all of these effects respond to oestrogen treatment and may improve a woman's sense of well-being during middle age. However, it should be recognized that HRT may postpone the natural processes of physiological adaptation to lower levels of oestrogen, and symptoms may reappear when treatment is withdrawn. A gradual attenuation of dosage may avoid this effect.

Other benefits may accrue from long-term HRT, but these require closer study and are definitely not yet indications for treatment. There is some evidence of protection from ischaemic heart disease (Hammond et al., 1979a; Ross et al., 1981). This could be attributed to a restoration of the blood lipid pattern of premenopause with lower serum cholesterol, of which a higher proportion is carried in the high-density lipoprotein fraction (Barrett-Connor et al., 1979; Nikkilä, 1978) (p. 138). Such findings may seem to conflict with the higher incidence of myocardial infarction among younger women using oral contraceptives (p. 117) and among men treated with oestrogen (Coronary Drug Project Research Group, 1970), although the preparations used are frequently different and of greater oestrogenic potency than those used in HRT. Oral contraceptives have been found to confer protection against rheumatoid arthritis (Royal College of General Practitioners' Oral Contraception Study, 1978), but it is doubtful whether this very minor effect is also conferred by HRT (World Health Organization, 1981).

7.2. How Is HRT Administered?

Natural oestrogens are most commonly used in administering HRT (e.g. oestradiol, oestrone, conjugated oestrogens), although synthetic forms are also available (e.g. ethinyl oestradiol), and even non-steroidal agents have been used (e.g. diethylstilboestrol). A detailed discussion of the clinical pharmacology of HRT is beyond the scope of this chapter, but a few pertinent biological facts will be outlined. The natural unconjugated steroid, oestradiol, is relatively inactive when administered orally, although activity is improved with "micronized" preparations. Oestrogen esters, such as those obtained from urine of pregnant mares (p. 18), are suitable alternatives as they are absorbed effectively from the gut. The oral route is preferred for administration of HRT but other routes are used, thus raising the oestradiol : oestrone ratio and minimizing effects on lipoprotein metabolism by avoiding the route involving the portal circulation and liver (Farish *et al.*, 1984). Oestrogen can be implanted or injected (e.g. oestradiol valerate), but these methods are time consuming and more difficult to control. Recently, oestradiol has been administered percutaneously in an ointment (Nichols *et al.*, 1984). The practice of using creams containing a natural oestrogen such as oestrone for topical application to the vaginal epithelium is well established. A smaller amount of oestrogen is then required than by the oral route, although a portion of it will be absorbed into the systemic circulation in sufficient quantities to have biological effects in other parts of the body (Punnonen *et al.*, 1980).

When protection against bone loss is required, oestrogen is frequently given in combination with other substances. The use of calcium and vitamin D will be mentioned shortly. Supplementary fluoride has also been found to be beneficial (Harrison *et al.*, 1981; Riggs *et al.*, 1982). This has the pharmacological effect of stimulating osteoblast activity rather than inhibiting bone resorption (Farley *et al.*, 1983).

The initiation and duration of treatment are matters requiring careful judgment and monitoring. Since the potential risks of therapy are likely to be dose related, it is prudent to use only the minimum dose required and for the shortest possible period for effective treatment and prophylaxis. As a further precaution, treatment is generally given cyclically to reduce undesirable stimulation of the endometrium. Interestingly, there is no biological reason *a priori* why treatment should mimic the 28-day cycle of premenopausal women, this being relatively rare among "primitive" hunter-gatherer societies, which have patterns of almost continuous pregnancy alternating with lactational amenorrhoea (Short, 1976).

7.3. What are the Risks of HRT?

A number of clinical conditions are aggravated by oestrogen treatment and so contraindicate the use of HRT, viz. history of thromboembolism, chronic liver disease, neuro-ophthalmological vascular disease, prophyria, endometriosis, oestrogen-dependent carcinoma of the genital tract or breast and undiagnosed vaginal bleeding (Edman, 1983). In addition, there is widespread concern that other women receiving HRT may have a higher risk of developing cardiovascular disease and cancer. Besides these fears, there is evidence of increased gallbladder disease (Boston Collaborative Drug Surveillance Program, 1974), but this has not been found in all surveys.

At present, the risks are mainly highlighted by epidemiological studies of younger women using oral contraceptives. However, it is not possible to ascertain precise risks because samples are not random and detection bias can arise (MacRae, 1981); besides, the doses used for older women are usually much lower than those used for contraception (e.g. 5–20μg cf. 30μg ethinyl oestradiol). Non-contraceptive oestrogens have been reported to increase the incidence of non-fatal myocardial infarction (Jick *et al.*, 1978b), but this has not been confirmed (Boston Collaborative Drug Surveillance Program, 1974; Pfeffer *et al.*, 1978). Synthetic hormones used in oral contraceptives affect blood-clotting factors (Meade, 1981), and, although treatment with natural oestrogen may not affect the coagulation–fibrinolysis system in the short-term (Notelovitz *et al.*, 1984), it is still a matter of concern whether HRT increases the risk of thrombosis. Whether natural oestrogens have the same undesirable effects as synthetic ones will not be discussed here, though it is worth reiterating that both desirable and undesirable effects are likely to be dose dependent (Hunter *et al.*, 1979). The risk of encouraging endometrial cancer cannot be estimated precisely for the same reasons as those given above for cardiovascular disease. However, it is recognized that continuous exposure to oestrogen unopposed is a factor and should be avoided if possible (British Gynaecological Cancer Group, 1981). Some workers suspect that the risk of breast cancer is also heightened by oestrogen exposure, but further evaluation is required before such claims are established (Hammond and Maxson, 1982; World Health Organization, 1981).

For these reasons, it is not advisable to use HRT overactively or indiscriminately. Most authorities now recommend that oestrogen treatment be combined with a progestogen for at least 10 days during the second half of a treatment cycle, except in hysterectomized women in whom combined treatment is not indicated (British Gynaecological Cancer Group, 1981). The addition of a progestogen does not seem to oppose the beneficial effects of oestrogen and may even reinforce them (Hammond *et al.*, 1979b). This can, of course, lead to regular vaginal bleeding, but it is a reassuring indication that any premalignant changes are being eliminated. It has been recommended that postmenopausal women, irrespective of whether they are receiving HRT, have an annual "progestogen challenge test" whilst risks of developing endometrial carcinoma from unopposed stimulation by oestrogen remain (Gambrell *et al.*, 1980). Withdrawal bleeding signals the need to continue providing progestogen during each cycle until this response disappears.

Despite the uncertain degree of risk associated with the use of HRT, it would seem prudent at the present time to minimize it by careful selection and monitoring of patients for the presence of cardiovascular disease and cancer. Progress towards identifying such risks by epidemiological studies is likely to be slow and controversial because of inherent limitations of methodology. A better understanding is likely to be obtained in the longer term by basic research into the biological mechanisms of oestrogen action.

7.4. Are There Alternatives to HRT?

Alternative forms of treatment for climacteric and postmenopausal complaints should be sought because exogenous oestrogen is contraindicated in some women and adverse publicity has raised concern about risks for others. Not all symptoms associated with menopause are related directly to withdrawal of oestrogen (e.g. depression), and other types of medication and/or counselling may be more appropriate. There are also prospects of eventually finding alternative treatments for vasomotor disturbances and postmenopausal bone loss, since the effects of oestrogen withdrawal on non-genital tissues appear to be indirect. However, at the present time alternatives to oestrogen for the treatment of these effects are generally less effective (e.g. calcitonin, clonidine) or may have undesirable side effects (e.g. androgens, progestogens). In the case of atrophy of the genito-urinary tract, it is unlikely that alternatives will be found since for epithelial growth it is necessary for cytosolic oestrogen receptors to be activated.

It is worth considering whether endogenous oestrogen levels can be bolstered to avoid the need for exogenous hormones altogether. White adipose tissue is capable of increasing the production of oestrogen from androstenedione, and a larger proportion of the product circulates in the unbound (biologically active) form in obese women (p. 33). Severe weight loss aggravates a low oestrogen status (O'Dea *et al.*, 1979). However, it would be unwise to advocate excessive weight gain in order to improve oestrogen status because the risks of a number of other diseases would be raised correspondingly. Moreover, it does not necessarily follow that obese women have fewer or less-severe climacteric symptoms (Hagen *et al.*, 1982b).

In principle, it should be possible to raise endogenous oestrogen levels by reducing the amount excreted in faeces. The intestinal microflora evidently play a major role in the entero-hepatic circulation by hydrolysing steroid conjugates, for when they are affected by administering antibiotics, less oestrogen is reabsorbed (Aldercreutz *et al.*, 1977; Back *et al.*, 1981) (p. 34). When rats were switched from a diet of grain to one containing meat, the levels of faecal β-glucuronidase were raised (Goldin and Gorbach, 1976). This effect, which probably reflects a changing microbial population in the gut, would be expeced to increase the hydrolysis and reabsorption of oestrogen glucuronides arriving via the bile duct. In women on a vegetarian diet, the amounts of oestrogen eliminated in the stool were increased threefold and the amounts of circulating oestrogen were reduced compared with omnivores, who lost more oestrogen in urine (Goldin *et al.*, 1981). In another study, there was no change in peripheral blood levels of oestrogen when postmenopausal women switched diets (Hill *et al.*, 1980). At present, there is insufficient evidence on which to base dietary control of hormone levels, and further research is needed to clarify these conflicting claims.

In contrast to these uncertainties, dietary calcium is a factor of major significance for the prophylaxis of bone loss. Calcium requirements rise with age, and a strong case has been made for increasing its intake in postmenopausal women who are in negative calcium balance (Dixon, 1983; Parfitt, 1983). The daily calcium requirement is the lowest intake necessary to maintain zero calcium balance in the majority of women (>95%). The requirement of premenopausal women aged 35–50 is 25 mmoles (1 g), whereas in older women it rises to 37.5 mmoles (1.5 g) (Heaney et al., 1978a). These figures are considerably higher than the currently recommended dietary allowances in the United Kingdom and the United States of 12.5 and 20 mmoles, respectively. Therefore, a supplement of at least 1 g of elemental calcium per day is likely to benefit women of postmenopausal age without significant risks of side effects. Supplementary calcium probably protects bones by a different mechanism to oestrogen. Increased absorption will reduce the levels of parathyroid hormone and 1,25-dihydroxycholecalciferol, in contrast to oestrogen, which increases production of the latter (p. 137). Calcium is frequently recommended in combination with either or both vitamin D and oestrogen, depending on whether the hormone is contraindicated and the severity of actual or potential bone loss (Nordin et al., 1980b; Gallagher et al., 1982). However, supplements of calcium with vitamin D may not conserve bone quite as effectively as oestrogen (Recker et al., 1977), and vitamin D should not be used alone because of the possibility of accelerating the demineralization of bone (Nordin et al., 1980a).

Physical exercise is another strategy for maintaining bone condition. When the normal stresses on the skeleton are removed, as in patients confined to bed and in astronauts during space flight, bone mineral is lost at a greater rate than in postmenopause (Bortz, 1982; Krølner and Toft, 1983). Resumption of normal regular activity reverses these changes, and even among animals exercise has been found to promote deposition of calcium in bone (LeBlanc et al., 1983). It is likely, therefore, that postmenopausal women would benefit from regular light exercise, which might not only reduce the risk of fractures by strengthening bone but also improve muscle tone and increase neuromuscular coordination (Twomey and Taylor, 1983). Exercise can also be recommended on other grounds, such as the raising of high density lipoprotein cholesterol, which may reduce atherogenesis (Cauley et al., 1982).

Vitamin E has sometimes been used for treating climacteric symptoms. This practice may have arisen from the early discovery that this vitamin is required for fertility in rats; indeed, its chemical name (d-α-tocopherol) means "oil of fertility" (Kitabchi, 1980). However, it is not known to be required for fertility in our own species, and a clinical deficiency state is not recognised. Vitamin E is known mainly by its anti-oxidant effects, and like other vitamins, it lacks oestrogenic activity. When the effects of vitamin E on climacteric symptoms were tested, the benefits were not significantly greater than those of placebos (Blatt *et al.*, 1953; Kupperman *et al.*, 1959), and current interest has now turned to the question of whether supplements can improve blood circulation (Hermann, 1982).

Finally, the fact that many women of middle age seek relief from their symptoms from sources outside medical and scientific orthodoxy should not be overlooked. In 1984, medical herbalists in Edinburgh enjoyed an active trade in remedies for the climacteric, but their customers may not have been aware that many preparations have attributes suggesting a connection with the ancient and discredited Doctrine of Signatures. This doctrine, which was raised to the status of an accepted science by Paracelsus (1493–1541), teaches that sympathetic interactions occur between substances and that, since plants were designed by their Creator for man, each carries a character or sign pointing to a special use. This would seem to explain why many contemporary herbal remedies for climacteric complaints are obtained from plants characterized either by late fragrance or red petals: oil of evening primrose (*Oenothera* spp.), centaury (*Centarium* spp.), vervain and other Verbenaceae. Such remedies should not, however, be dismissed lightly, and careful, controlled studies of their properties might be worthwhile. Whilst their effects may turn out to be no better than those of placebos, they are nevertheless valuable, as are the laxative and carminative properties, vitamins and trace elements that herbs can provide. In other parts of the world, the use of herbal remedies is even more widespread. In the Peoples' Republic of China, herbal medicine is dispensed side by side with modern drugs, and is presently under laboratory investigation at the respected Research Institute of Traditional Medicine in Beijing and elsewhere. The natural materials are obtained from seeds, flowers and roots, which are infused to make a drink (Xiao Bilian, personal communication). Whilst opinions of the efficacy of these materials must be reserved until further information is available, the use of alternative treatments for the climacteric in different parts of the world serves to illustrate an almost universal interest in the manifestations of the ageing reproductive system.

References

Abraham, G. E. (1974). Ovarian and adrenal contribution to peripheral androgens during the menstrual cycle. *J. Clin. Endocrinol. Metab.* **39**, 340–346.

Abraham, G. E. and Maroulis, G. B. (1975). Effect of exogenous estrogen on serum pregnenolone, cortisol and androgens in postmenopausal women. *Obstet. Gynecol.* **45**, 271–274.

Abramson, J. H., Gampel, B., Slome, C. and Scotch, N. (1960). Age at menopause of urban Zulu women. *Science* **132**, 356–357.

Adams, C. E. (1970). Ageing and reproduction in the female mammal with particular reference to the rabbit. *J. Reprod. Fertil. Suppl.* **12**, 1–16.

Aiyer, M. S., Fink, G. and Greig, F. (1974). Changes in the sensitivity of the pituitary gland to luteinizing hormone releasing factor during the oestrous cycle of the rat. *J. Endocrinol.* **60**, 47–64.

Aksel, S., Schomberg, D. W., Tyrey, L. and Hammond, C. B. (1976). Vasomotor symptoms, serum estrogens, and gonadotropin levels in surgical menopause. *Am. J. Obstet. Gynecol.* **126**, 165–169.

Alberman, E., Creasy, M., Elliott, M. and Spicer, C. (1976). Maternal factors associated with fetal chromosomal anomalies in spontaneous abortions. *Br. J. Obstet. Gynaecol.* **83**, 621–627.

Albright, F., Smith, P. H. and Richardson, A. M. (1941). Postmenopausal osteoporosis: Its clinical features. *JAMA, J. Am. Med. Assoc.* **116**, 2465–2474.

Aldercreutz, H., Martin, F., Lehtinen, T., Tikkanen, M. J. and Pulkkinen, M. O. (1977). Effect of ampicillin administration on plasma conjugated and unconjugated estrogen and progesterone levels in pregnancy. *Am. J. Obstet, Gynecol.* **128**, 266–271.

Allen, E. (1941). Glandular physiology and therapy. Physiology of the ovaries. *JAMA, J. Am. Med. Assoc.* **116**, 405–412.

Allen, E. and Doisy, E. A. (1923). An ovarian hormone. Preliminary report on its localization, extraction and partial purification, and action in test animals. *JAMA, J. Am. Med. Assoc.* **81**, 819–821.

Ames, S. R. (1974). Age, parity and vitamin A supplementation and the vitamin E requirement of female rats. *Am. J. Clin. Nutr.* **27**, 1017–1025.

Amundsen, D. W. and Diers, C. J. (1970). The age of menopause in classical Greece and Rome. *Hum. Biol.* **42**, 79–86.

Amundsen, D. W. and Diers, C. J. (1973). The age of menopause in Mediaeval Europe. *Hum. Biol.* **45**, 605–612.

Anderson, J. N., Peck, E. J., Jr. and Clark, J. H. (1975). Estrogen-induced uterine responses and growth: Relationship to receptor estrogen binding by uterine nuclei. *Endocrinology* **96**, 160–167.

Angell, R. R., Aitken, R. J., van Look, P. F. A., Lumsden, M. A. and Templeton, A. A. (1983). Chromosome abnormalities in human embryos after *in vitro* fertilization. *Nature (London)* **303**, 336–338.

Armstrong, D. T. and Papkoff, H. (1976). Stimulation of aromatization of exogenous and endogenous androgens in ovaries of hypophysectomized rats *in vivo* by follicle-stimulating hormone. *Endocrinology* **99**, 1144–1151.

Armstrong, D. T., Goff, A. K. and Dorrington, J. H. (1979). Regulation of follicular estrogen biosynthesis. *In* "Ovarian Follicular Development and Function" (A. R. Midgley and W. A. Sadler, eds.), pp. 169–181. Raven Press, New York.

Aschheim, P. (1964–1965). Résultats fournis par la greffe hétérochrone des ovaries dans l'étude de la régulation hypothalamo-hypophyso-ovarienne de la ratte sénile. *Gerontologia* **10**, 65–75.

Aschheim, P. (1976). Aging in the hypothalamic-hypophyseal ovarian axis in the rat. *In* "Hypothalamus, Pituitary and Aging" (A. V. Everitt and J. A. Burgess, eds.), pp. 376–418. Thomas, Springfield, Illinois.

Asdell, S. A., Bogart, R. and Sperling, G. (1941). The influence of age and rate of breeding upon the ability of the female rat to reproduce and raise young. *Mem. N.Y., Agric. Exp. Stn. (Ithaca)* **238**, 1–26.

Atkins, D., Zanelli, J. M., Peacock, M. and Nordin, B. E. C. (1972). The effect of oestrogens on the response of bone to parathyroid hormone *in vitro*. *J. Endocrinol.* **54**, 107–117.

Austin, C. R. (1970). Ageing and reproduction: Post-ovulatory deterioration of the egg. *J. Reprod. Fertil., Suppl.* **12**, 39–53.

Aymé, S. and Lippman-Hand, A. (1982). Maternal-age effect in aneuploidy: Does altered embryonic selection play a role? *Am. J. Hum. Genet.* **34**, 558–565.

Back, D. J., Chapman, C. R., May, S. A. and Rowe, P. H. (1981). Absorption of oestrone sulphate from the gastrointestinal tract of the rat. *J. Steroid Biochem.* **14**, 347–356.

Backman, G. (1948). Die Beschleunigte Entwicklung der Jugend. *Acta Anat.* **4**, 421–480.

Bäckström, C. T., McNeilly, A. S., Leask, R. M. and Baird, D. T. (1982). Pulsatile secretion of LH, FSH, prolactin, oestradiol and progesterone during the human menstrual cycle. *Clin. Endocrinol. (Oxford)* **17**, 29–42.

Badawy, S. Z. A., Elliott, L. J., Elbadawi, A. and Marshall, L. D. (1979). Plasma levels of oestrone and oestradiol-17β in postmenopausal women. *Br. J. Obstet. Gynaecol.* **86**, 56–63.

Baird, D. T. (1977a). Evidence *in vivo* for the two-cell hypothesis of oestrogen synthesis by the sheep Graafian follicle. *J. Reprod. Fertil.* **50**, 183–185.

Baird, D. T. (1977b). Synthesis and secretion of steroid hormones by the ovary *in vivo*. *In* "The Ovary" (L. Zuckerman and B. J. Weir, eds.), 2nd ed., Vol. 3, pp. 305–357. Academic Press, New York.

Baird, D. T. (1983). Factors regulating the growth of the preovulatory follicle in the sheep and human. *J. Reprod. Fertil.* **69**, 343–352.

Baird, D. T. and Fraser, I. S. (1974). Blood production and ovarian secretion rates of estradiol-17β and estrone in women throughout the menstrual cycle. *J. Clin. Endocrinol. Metab.* **38**, 1009–1017.

Baird, D. T. and Guevara, A. (1969). Concentrations of unconjugated estrone and estradiol in peripheral plasma in non-pregnant women throughout the menstrual cycle, castrate and postmenopausal women and in men. *J. Clin. Endocrinol. Metab.* **29**, 149–156.

Baird, D. T., Uno, A. and Melby, J. C. (1969). Adrenal secretion of androgens and oestrogens. *J. Endocrinol.* **45**, 135–136.

Baird, D. T., Burger, P. E., Heavon-Jones, G. D. and Scaramuzzi, R. J. (1974). The site of secretion of androstenedione in non-pregnant women. *J. Endocrinol.* **63**, 201–212.

Baker, T. G. (1963). A quantitative and cytological study of germ cells in human ovaries. *Proc. R. Soc. London, Ser. B* **158**, 417–433.

Baker, T. G. (1971). Radiosensitivity of mammalian oocytes with particular reference to the human female. *Am. J. Obstet. Gynecol.* **110**, 746–761.

Baker, T. G. and McLaren, A. (1973). The effect of tritiated thymidine on the developing oocytes of mice. *J. Reprod. Fertil.* **34**, 121–130.

Baker, T. G. and Neal, P. (1974). Oogenesis in human fetal ovaries maintained in organ culture. *J. Anat.* **117**, 591–604.

Baker, T. G. and Neal, P. (1977). Action of ionizing radiations on the mammalian ovary. *In* "The Ovary" (L. Zuckerman and B. J. Weir, eds.), 2nd ed., Vol. 3, pp. 1–58. Academic Press, New York.

Baker, T. G. and Scrimgeour, J. B. (1980). Development of the gonad in normal and anencephalic human fetuses. *J. Reprod. Fertil.* **60**, 193–199.

Baker, T. G., Challoner, S. and Burgoyne, P. S. (1980). The number of oocytes in unilaterally overiectomized mice up to 8 months after surgery. *J. Reprod. Fertil.* **60**, 449–456.

Ball, P., Knuppen, R., Haupt, M. and Breuer, H. (1972). Interactions between estrogens and catechol amines. III. Studies on the methylation of catechol estrogens, catechol amines and other catechols by the catechol-O-methyltransferase of human liver. *J. Clin. Endocrinol. Metab.* **34**, 736–746.

Bancroft, J. D. (1983). "Human Sexuality and its Problems." Churchill-Livingstone, Edinburgh and London.

Barlow, J. J., Emerson, K., Jr. and Saxena, B. N. (1969). Estradiol production after ovariectomy for carcinoma of the breast. *N. Engl. J. Med.* **280**, 633–637.

Barr, D. P. (1953). Some chemical factors in the pathogenesis of atherosclerosis. *Circulation* **8**, 641–654.

Barrett-Connor, E., Brown, W. V., Turner, J., Austin, M. and Criqui, M. H. (1979). Heart disease risk factors and hormone use in postmenopausal women. *JAMA, J. Am. Med. Assoc.* **241**, 2167–2169.

Baschieri, L., Martino, E., Mariotti, S., Lippi, F., Monzani, F., Motz, E., Vaudagna, G. and Aloisio, V. (1982). Thyroid and menopause. *In* "The Menopause: Clinical, Endocrinological and Pathophysiological Aspects" (P. Fioretti, L. Martini, G. B. Melis and S. S. C. Yen, eds.), Serono Found. Symp. 39, pp. 179–188. Academic Press, New York.

Batta, S. K., Wentz, A. C. and Channing, C. P. (1980). Steroidogenesis by human ovarian cell types in culture: Influence of mixing of cell types and effect of added testosterone. *J. Clin. Endocrinol. Metab.* **50**, 274–279.

Bean, J. A., Leeper, J. D., Wallace, R. B., Sherman, B. M. and Jagger, H. (1979). Variations in the reporting of menstrual histories. *Am. J. Epidemiol.* **109**, 181–185.

Beatty, R. A. (1958). Variation in the number of corpora lutea and in the number and size of 6-day blastocysts in rabbits subjected to superovulation treatment. *J. Endocrinol.* **17**, 248–260.

Beaumont, H. M. and Mandl, A. M. (1962). A quantitative and cytological study of oogonia and oocytes in the foetal and neonatal rat. *Proc. R. Soc. London, Ser. B* **155**, 557–579.

Belisle, S., Beaudry, C. and Lehoux, J.-G. (1982). Endocrine aging in CBA mice: Characterization of uterine cytosolic and nuclear sex steroid receptors. *Exp. Gerontol.* **17**, 417–423.

Benedetti, W. L., Sala, M. A. and Otegui, J. T. (1976). Persistent estrus in rats after anterolateral hypothalamic microinjections of 6-hydroxydopamine. *Neuroendocrinology* **21**, 297–303.

Bengtsson, C. (1979). Is the menopausal age rapidly changing? *Maturitas* **1**, 159–164.

Bengtsson, C., Lindquist, O. and Redvall, L. (1981). Menstrual status and menopausal age of middle-aged Swedish women. *Acta Obstet. Gynecol. Scand.* **60**, 269–275.

Benjamin, F. (1960). The age of the menarche and of the menopause in white South African women and certain factors influencing these times. *S. Afr. Med. J.* **34**, 316–320.

Biggers, J. D. (1976). General principles of contraceptive technology. *In* "Regulation of Human Fertility" (K. S. Moghissi and T. N. Evans, eds.), pp. 28–56. Wayne State Univ. Press, Detroit, Michigan.

Biggers, J. D., Finn, C. A. and McLaren, A. (1962). Long-term reproductive performance of female mice. II. Variation of litter size with parity. *J. Reprod. Fertil.* **3**, 313–330.

Billewicz, W. Z. (1973). Some implications of self-selection for pregnancy. *Br. J. Prev. Soc. Med.* **27**, 49–52.

Blaha, G. C. (1964). Effect of age of the donor and recipient on the development of transferred golden hamster ova. *Anat. Rec.* **150**, 413–416.

Blaha, G. C. and Leavitt, W. W. (1978). Uterine progesterone receptors in the aged golden hamster. *J. Gerontol.* **33**, 810–814.

Blake, C. A., Weiner, R. I., Gorski, R. A. and Sawyer, C. H. (1972). Secretion of pituitary luteinizing hormone and follicle stimulating hormone in female rats made persistently estrous or diestrous by hypothalamic deafferentation. *Endocrinology* **90**, 855–861.

Blake, C. A., Elias, K. A. and Huffman, L. J. (1983). Ovariectomy of young adult rats has a sparing effect on the ability of aged rats to release luteinizing hormone. *Biol. Reprod.* **28**, 575–585.

Blatt, M. H. G., Wiesbader, H. and Kupperman, H. S. (1953). Vitamin E and climacteric syndrome. *Arch. Intern. Med.* **91**, 792–799.

Bloch, K. (1945). The biological conversion of cholesterol to pregnanediol. *J. Biol. Chem.* **157**, 661–666.

Bloch, S. and Flury, E. (1959). Untersuchungen über Klimakterium und Menopause an Albino-Ratten. *Gynaecologia* **147**, 414–438.

Block, E. (1952). Quantitative morphological investigations of the follicular system in women. *Acta Anat.* **14**, 108–123.

Bogovich, K. and Richards, J. S. (1982). Androgen biosynthesis in developing ovarian follicles: Evidence that luteinizing hormone regulates thecal 17-hydroxylase and $C_{17\text{-}20}$-lyase activities. *Endocrinology* **111**, 1201–1208.

Bond, D. J. and Chandley, A. C. (1983). "Aneuploidy." Oxford Univ. Press, London and New York.

Bongaarts, J. (1980). Does malnutrition affect fecundity? A summary of evidence. *Science* **208**, 564–569.

Bongaarts, J. (1982). Infertility after age 30: A false alarm. *Fam. Plann. Perspect.* **14**, 75–78.

Bortz, W. M., II (1982). Disuse and aging. *JAMA, J. Am. Med. Assoc.* **248**, 1203–1208.

Boston Collaborative Drug Surveillance Program (1974). Surgically confirmed gallbladder disease, venous thromboembolism, and breast tumours in relation to postmenopausal estrogen therapy. *N. Engl. J. Med.* **290**, 15–19.

Boué, J., Boué, A. and Lazar, P. (1975). The epidemiology of human spontaneous abortions with chromosomal anomalies. *In* "Aging Gametes" (R. J. Blandau, ed.), pp. 330–348. Karger, Basel.

Brand, P. C. and Lehert, P. (1978). A new way of looking at environmental variables that may affect the age at menopause. *Maturitas* **1**, 121–132.

Braw, R. H. and Tsafriri, A. (1980a). Follicles explanted from pentobarbitone-treated rats provide a model for atresia. *J. Reprod. Fertil.* **59**, 259–265.

Braw, R. H. and Tsafriri, A. (1980b). Effect of PMSG on follicular atresia in the immature rat ovary. *J. Reprod. Fertil.* **59**, 267–272.

Braw, R. H., Bar-Ami, S. and Tsafriri, A. (1981). Effect of hypophysectomy on atresia of rat preovulatory follicles. *Biol. Reprod.* **25**, 989–996.

Brawer, J. R., Naftolin, F., Martin, J. and Sonenschein, C. (1978). Effects of a single injection of estradiol valerate on the hypothalamic arcuate nucleus and on reproductive function in the female rat. *Endocrinology* **103**, 501–512.

Brawer, J. R., Schipper, H. and Naftolin, F. (1980). Ovary-dependent degeneration in the hypothalamic arcuate nucleus. *Endocrinology* **107**, 274–279.

British Gynaecological Cancer Group (1981). Oestrogen replacement and endometrial cancer. *Lancet* **1,** 1359–1360.

Brook, J. D., Gosden, R. G. and Chandley, A. C. (1984). Maternal ageing and aneuploid embryos: Evidence from the mouse that biological and not chronological age is the important influence. *Hum. Genet.* **66,** 41–45.

Broom, T. J., Matthews, C. D., Cooke, I. D., Ralph, M. M., Seamark, R. F. and Cox, L. W. (1981). Endocrine profiles and fertility status of human menstrual cycles of varying follicular phase length. *Fertil. Steril.* **36,** 194–200.

Brown, C., Gosden, R. G. and Poyser, N. L. (1984). Effects of age and steroid treatment on prostaglandin production by the rat uterus in relation to implantation. *J. Reprod. Fertil.* **70,** 649–656.

Brown, J. B. (1978). Pituitary control of ovarian function-concepts derived from gonadotrophin therapy. *Aust. N.Z. J. Obstet. Gynaecol.* **18,** 47–54.

Bullough, H. F. (1947). Epidermal thickness following oestrone injections in the mouse. *Nature (London)* **159,** 101–102.

Bulmer, M. G. (1970). "The Biology of Twinning in Man." Oxford Univ. Press (Clarendon), London and New York.

Burch, P. R. J. and Gunz, F. W. (1967). The distribution of menopausal age in New Zealand. An exploratory study. *N.Z. Med. J.* **66,** 6–10.

Burgoyne, P. S. and Baker, T. G. (1981a). Oocyte depletion in XO mice and their XX sibs from 12 to 200 days post partum. *J. Reprod. Fertil.* **61,** 207–212.

Burgoyne, P. S. and Baker, T. G. (1981b). The XO ovary-development and function. *In* "Development and Function of Reproductive Organs" (A. G. Byskov and H. Peters, eds.), I.C.S. No. 559, pp. 122–128. Excerpta Medica, Amsterdam.

Burton, R. M. and Westphal, U. (1972). Steroid hormone-binding proteins in blood plasma. *Metab., Clin. Exp.* **21,** 253–276.

Butcher, R. L. and Fugo, N. W. (1967). Overripeness and mammalian ova. II. Delayed ovulation and chromosome anomalies. *Fertil. Steril.* **18,** 297–302.

Butcher, R. L. and Pope, R. S. (1979). Role of estrogen during prolonged estrous cycles of the rat on subsequent embryonic death or development. *Biol. Reprod.* **21,** 491–495.

Butenandt, A. and Westphal, U. (1974). Isolation of progesterone - forty years ago. *Am. J. Obstet. Gynecol.* **120,** 138–141.

Byskov, A. G. S. (1974). Cell kinetic studies of follicular atresia in the mouse ovary. *J. Reprod. Fertil.* **37,** 277–285.

Byskov, A. G. S. (1975). The role of the rete ovarii in meiosis and follicle formation in the cat, mink and ferret. *J. Reprod. Fertil.* **45,** 201–209.

Calanog, A., Sall, S., Gordon, G. G. and Southren, A. L. (1977). Androstenedione metabolism in patients with endometrial cancer. *Am. J. Obstet. Gynecol.* **129,** 553–556.

Campbell, S. (1976). Intensive steroid and protein hormone profiles on post-menopausal women experiencing hot flushes, and a group of controls. *In* "The Management of the Menopause and Post-menopausal Years" (S. Campbell, ed.), pp. 63–77. MTP Press, Lancaster.

Cannings, C. and Cannings, M. R. (1968). Mongolism, delayed fertilization and human sexual behaviour. *Nature (London)* **218,** 481.

Cannon, W. B. (1932). "The Wisdom of the Body." Kegan Paul, Trench, Trubner & Co., Ltd., London.

Carothers, A. D. (1983). Evidence that altered embryonic selection contributes to maternal age effect in aneuploidy: A spurious conclusion attributable to pooling of heterogeneous data? *Am. J. Hum. Genet.* **35,** 1057–1059.

Carr, D. H., Haggar, R. A. and Hart, A. G. (1968). Germ cells in the ovaries of XO female infants. *Am. J. Clin. Pathol.* **49,** 521–526.

Carson, R. S., Findlay, J. K., Burger, H. G. and Trounson, A. O. (1979). Gonadotropin receptors of the ovine ovarian follicle during follicular growth and atresia. *Biol. Reprod.* **21**, 75–87.

Carter, C. O. and Evans, K. (1973). Spina bifida and anencephalus in Greater London. *J. Med. Genet.* **10**, 209–234.

Carter, C. O., David, P. A. and Laurence, K. M. (1968). A family study of major central nervous system malformations in South Wales. *J. Med. Genet.* **5**, 81–106.

Casper, R. F. and Yen, S. S. C. (1981). Menopausal flushes: Effect of pituitary gonadotropin desensitization by a potent luteinizing hormone-releasing factor agonist. *J. Clin. Endocrinol. Metab.* **53**, 1056–1058.

Casper, R. F., Yen, S. S. C. and Wilkes, M. M. (1979). Menopausal flushes: A neuroendocrine link with pulsatile luteinizing hormone secretion. *Science* **205**, 823–825.

Catherwood, B. D., Omishi, T. and Deftos, L. J. (1983). Effect of estrogens and phosphorus depletion on plasma calcitonin in the rat. *Calcif. Tissue Int.* **35**, 502–507.

Cauley, J. A., La Porte, R. E., Kuller, L. H. and Black-Sandler, R. (1982). The epidemiology of high density lipoprotein cholesterol levels in post-menopausal women. *J. Gerontol.* **37**, 10–15.

Chakravarti, S., Collins, W. P., Forecast, J. D., Newton, J. R., Oram, D. H. and Studd, J. W. W. (1976). Hormonal profiles after the menopause. *Br. Med. J.* **2**, 784–787.

Chakravarti, S., Collins, W. P., Newton, J. R., Oram, D. H. and Studd, J. W. W. (1977). Endocrine changes and symptomatology after oophorectomy in premenopausal women. *Br. J. Obstet. Gynaecol.* **84**, 769–775.

Chakravarti, S., Collins, W. P., Thom, M. H. and Studd, J. W. W. (1979). Relation between plasma hormone profiles, symptoms, and response to oestrogen treatment in women approaching the menopause. *Br. Med. J.* **1**, 983–985.

Channing, C. P. and Coudert, S. P. (1976). Contribution of granulosa cells and follicular fluid to ovarian estrogen secretion in the rhesus monkey *in vivo. Endocrinology* **98**, 590–597.

Chatterjee, A. and Greenwald, G. S. (1972). The long-term effects of unilateral ovariectomy of the cycling hamster and rat. *Biol. Reprod.* **7**, 238–246.

Chavez, A. and Martinez, C. (1982). "Growing up in a Developing Community." Institute of Nutrition of Central America and Panama, Mexico.

Chen, T. L. and Feldman, D. (1978). Distinction between alpha-fetoprotein and intracellular estrogen receptors: Evidence against the presence of estradiol receptors in rat bone. *Endocrinology* **102**, 236–244.

Chen, Y.-T., Mattison, D. R., Feigenbaum, L., Fukui, H. and Schulman, J. D. (1981). Reduction in oocyte number following prenatal exposure to a diet high in galactose. *Science* **214**, 1145–1147.

Chestnut, C. H., Baylink, D. J., Sisom, K., Nelp, W. B. and Roos, B. A. (1980). Basal plasma immunoreactive calcitonin in postmenopausal osteoporosis. *Metab., Clin. Exp.* **29**, 559–562.

Christiansen, C., Mazess, R. B., Transbøl, I. and Jensen, G. F. (1981). Factors in response to treatment of early postmenopausal bone loss. *Calcif. Tissue Int.* **33**, 575–581.

Christiansen, C., Christensen, M. S., Larsen, N.-E. and Transbøl, I. (1982). Pathophysiological mechanisms of estrogen effect on bone metabolism. Dose-response relationships in early postmenopausal woman. *J. Clin. Endocrinol. Metab.* **55**, 1124–1130.

Clarke, I. J. and Cummins, J. T. (1982). The temporal relationship between gonadotropin releasing hormone (GnRH) and luteinizing hormone secretion in ovariectomized ewes. *Endocrinology* **111**, 1737–1739.

Clayden, J. R., Bell, J. W. and Pollard, P. (1974). Menopausal flushing: double-blind trial of a non-hormonal medication. *Br. Med. J.* **1**, 409–412.

Clos, J. A. (1858). De l'influence de la lune sur la menstruation. *Bull. Cl. Sci., Acad. R. Sci. Belg.* [2] **4**, 108–160.

Coble, Y. D., Jr., Kohler, P. O., Cargille, C. M. and Ross, G. T. (1969). Production rates and metabolic clearance rates of human follicle-stimulating hormone in premenopausal and postmenopausal women. *J. Clin. Invest.* **48,** 359–363.

Cohn, S. H. (1980). The present state of *in vivo* neutron activation analysis in clinical diagnosis and therapy. *At. Energy Rev.* **18,** 599–660.

Cohn, S. H., Vaswani, A., Zanzi, I., Aloia, J. F., Roginsky, M. S. and Ellis, K. J. (1976). Changes in body chemical composition with age measured by total-body neutron activation. *Metab., Clin. Exp.* **25,** 85–95.

Cohn, S. H., Abesamis, C., Zanzi, I., Aloia, J. F., Yasumura, S. and Ellis, K. J. (1977). Body elemental composition: Comparison between black and white adults. *Am. J. Physiol.* **232,** E419–E422.

Collett, M. E., Wertenberger, G. E. and Fiske, V. M. (1954). The effect of age upon the pattern of the menstrual cycle. *Fertil. Steril.* **5,** 437–448.

Collman, R. D. and Stoller, A. (1962). A survey of mongoloid births in Victoria, Australia, 1942–1957. *Am. J. Public Health* **52,** 813–829.

Cooper, R. L. and Linnoila, M. (1977). Sexual behaviour in aged, non-cycling female rats. *Physiol. Behav.* **18,** 573–576.

Cooper, R. L. and Linnoila, M. (1980). Effects of centrally and systemically administered L-tyrosine and L-leucine on ovarian function in the old rat. *Gerontology* **26,** 270–275.

Cooper, R. L., Conn, P. M. and Walker, R. F. (1980). Characterization of the LH surge in middle-aged female rats. *Biol. Reprod.* **23,** 611–615.

Cooper, R. L., Roberts, B., Rogers, D. C., Seay, S. G. and Conn, P. M. (1984). Endocrine status *versus* chronologic age as predictors of altered luteinizing hormone secretion in the "aging" rat. *Endocrinology* **114,** 391–396.

Coronary Drug Project Research Group (1970). The coronary drug project: Initial findings leading to modifications of its research protocol. *JAMA, J. Am. Med. Assoc.* **214,** 1303–1313.

Costoff, A. and Mahesh, V. B. (1975). Primordial follicles with normal oocytes in the ovaries of postmenopausal women. *J. Am. Geriatr. Soc.* **23,** 193–196.

Coulam, C. B. and Ryan, R. J. (1979). Premature menopause. I. Etiology. *Am. J. Obstet. Gynecol.* **133,** 639–643.

Court Brown, W. M., Law, P. and Smith, P. G. (1969). Sex chromosome aneuploidy and parental age. *Ann. Hum. Genet.* **33,** 1–14.

Crilly, R. G., Marshall, D. H. and Nordin, B. E. C. (1979). Effect of age on plasma androstenedione concentration in oophorectomized women. *Clin. Endocrinol. (Oxford)* **10,** 199–201.

Crilly, R. G., Francis, R. M. and Nordin, B. E. C. (1981). Steroid hormones, ageing and bone. *Clin. Endocrinol. Metab.* **10,** 115–139.

Crowley, P. H., Gulati, D. K., Hayden, T. L., Lopez, P. and Dyer, R. (1979). A chiasma-hormonal hypothesis relating Down's syndrome and maternal age. *Nature (London)*, **280,** 417–419.

Crumeyrolle-Arias, M. and Aschheim, P. (1981). Post-hypophysectomy ovarian senescence and its relation to the spontaneous structural changes in the ovary of intact aged rats. *Gerontology* **27,** 58–71.

Crumeyrolle-Arias, M., Scheib, D. and Aschheim, P. (1976). Light and electron microscopy of the ovarian interstitial tissue in the senile rat: Normal aspect and response to HCG of "deficiency cells" and "epithelial cords." *Gerontology* **22,** 185–204.

Csapo, A. I., Pulkkinen, M. O. and Kaihola, H. L. (1974). The relationship between the timing of luteectomy and the incidence of complete abortions. *Am. J. Obstet. Gynecol.* **118,** 985–989.

Daniell, H. W. (1976). Osteoporosis of the slender smoker. *Arch. Intern. Med.* **136,** 298–304.

Dao, T.L.-Y. (1953). Estrogen excretion in women with mammary cancer before and after adrenalectomy. *Science* **118,** 21–22.

Davidge, J. B. (1814). Menstruous action. *In* "Physical Sketches, or Outlines of Correctives,

Applied to Certain Modern Errours in Physick," pp. 31–56. Warner & Robinson, Baltimore, Maryland.

Davidson, B. J., Ross, R. K., Paganini-Hill, A., Hammond, G. D., Siiteri, P. K. and Judd, H. L. (1982). Total and free estrogens and androgens in postmenopausal women with hip fractures. *J. Clin. Endocrinol. Metab.* **54**, 115–120.

Davidson, B. J., Riggs, B. L., Wahner, H. W. and Judd, H. L. (1983). Endogenous cortisol and sex steroids in patients with osteoporotic spinal fractures. *Obstet. Gynecol.* **61**, 275–278.

DeFazio, J., Meldrum, D. R., Laufer, L., Vale, W., Rivier, J., Lu, J. K. H. and Judd, H. L. (1983). Induction of hot flashes in premenopausal women treated with a long-acting GnRH agonist. *J. Clin. Endocrinol. Metab.* **56**, 445–448.

DeFazio, J., Verheugen, C., Chetkowski, R., Nass, T., Judd, H. L. and Meldrum, D. R. (1984). The effects of naloxone on hot flashes and gonadotropin secretion in postmenopausal women. *J. Clin. Endocrinol. Metab.* **58**, 578–581.

de Gardanne, C. P. L. (1816). "Avis aux femmes qui entrent dans l'âge critique." Paris.

de Jong, F. H. and Sharpe, R. M. (1976). Evidence for inhibin-like activity in bovine follicular fluid. *Nature* (*London*) **263**, 71–72.

de Jong, F. H., Baird, D. T. and van der Molen, H. J. (1974). Ovarian secretion rates of oestrogens, androgens and progesterone in normal women and in women with persistent ovarian follicles. *Acta Endocrinol.* (*Copenhagen*) **77**, 575–587.

Delmas, P. D., Stenner, D., Wahner, H. W., Mann, K. G. and Riggs, B. L. (1983). Increase in serum bone γ-carboxyglutamic acid protein with aging in women. *J. Clin. Invest.* **71**, 1316–1321.

de Moraes-Ruehsen, M., Blizzard, R. M., Garcia-Bunuel, R. and Jones, G. S. (1972). Autoimmunity and ovarian failure. *Am. J. Obstet. Gynecol.* **112**, 693–703.

Dennefors, B. L., Janson, P. O., Hamberger, L. and Knutsson, F. (1982). Hilus cells from human postmenopausal ovaries: Gonadotrophin sensitivity, steroid and cyclic AMP production. *Acta Obstet. Gynecol. Scand.* **61**, 413–416.

Dennerstein, L., Burrows, G. D., Hyman, G. and Wood, C. (1978). Menopausal hot flushes: A double blind comparison of placebo, ethinyl oestradiol and norgestrel. *Br. J. Obstet. Gynaecol.* **85**, 852–856.

Department of Health and Social Security (1982). "Report of Confidential Enquiries into Maternal Deaths in England and Wales, 1976–78." HMSO, London.

Dequecker, J., Remans, J., Franssen, R. and Waes, J. (1971). Ageing patterns of trabecular and cortical bone and their relationship. *Calcif. Tissue Res.* **7**, 23–30.

Diamond, I., Anderson, M. M. and McCreadie, S. R. (1960). Transplacental transmission of busulphan (Myleran) in a mother with leukemia. Production of fetal malformation and cytomegaly. *Pediatrics* **25**, 85–90.

Diamond, J. M. (1982). Big-bang reproduction and ageing in male marsupial mice. *Nature* (*London*) **298**, 115–116.

Dierschke, D. J., Koening, J., Krueger, G. and Robinson, J. A. (1983). Reproductive and hormonal patterns in perimenopausal rhesus monkeys. *Program Endocr. Soc.*, Abstr. No. 678.

Dietrich, A. J. J. and Mulder, R. J. P. (1983). A light and electron microscopic analysis of meiotic prophase in female mice. *Chromosoma* **88**, 377–385.

Dilman, V. M. (1971). Age-associated elevation of hypothalamic threshold to feedback control and its role in development, ageing and disease. *Lancet* **1**, 1211–1219.

Dixon, A. St. J. (1983). Non-hormonal treatment of osteoporosis. *Br. Med. J.* (286), 999–1000.

DiZerega, G. S., Marrs, R. P., Roche, P. C., Campeau, J. D. and Kling, O. R. (1983). Identification of proteins in pooled human follicular fluid which suppress follicular response to gonadotropins. *J. Clin. Endocrinol. Metab.* **56**, 35–41.

Dodds, E. C., Goldberg, L., Lawson, W. and Robinson, R. (1938). Oestrogenic activity of alkylated stilboestrols. *Nature (London)* **142,** 34.

Doisy, E. A. (1972). Isolation of a crystalline estrogen from urine and the follicular hormone from ovaries. *Am. J. Obstet. Gynecol.* **114,** 701–702.

Döring, G. K. (1963). Über die relative Häufigkeit des anovulatorischen cyclus im Leben der Frau. *Arch. Gynaekol.* **199,** 115–123.

Dorrington, J. H., Moon, Y. S. and Armstrong, D. T. (1975). Estradiol-17β bisynthesis in cultured granulosa cells from hypophysectomized immature rats; stimulation by follicle-stimulating hormone. *Endocrinology* **97,** 1328–1331.

Eaton, J. W. and Mayer, A. J. (1953). The social biology of very high fertility among the Hutterites. The demography of a unique population. *Hum. Biol.* **25,** 206–264.

Edman, C. D. (1983). Estrogen replacement therapy. *In* "The Menopause" (H. J. Buchsbaum, ed.), pp. 77–84. Springer-Verlag, Berlin and New York.

Edman, C. D., Aiman, E. J., Porter, J. C. and MacDonald, P. C. (1978). Identification of the estrogen product of extraglandular aromatization of plasma androstenedione. *Am. J. Obstet. Gynecol.* **130,** 439–447.

Edmonds, D. K., Lindsay, K. S., Miller, J. F., Williamson, E. and Wood, P. J. (1982). Early embryonic mortality in women. *Fertil. Steril.* **38,** 447–453.

Edwards, R. G. and Steptoe, P. C. (1983). Current status of *in vitro* fertilization and implantation of human embryos. *Lancet* **2,** 1265–1269.

Edwards, R. G., Steptoe, P. C., Abraham, G. E., Walters, E., Purdy, J. M. and Fotherby, K. (1972). Steroid assays and preovulatory follicular development in human ovaries primed with gonadotrophins. *Lancet* **2,** 611–615.

Epstein, C. J., Epstein, L. B., Weil, J. and Cox, D. R. (1982). Trisomy 21: Mechanisms and models. *Ann. N.Y. Acad. Sci.* **396,** 107–118.

Erickson, B. H., Reynolds, R. A. and Murphree, R. L. (1976). Ovarian characteristics and reproductive performance of the aged cow. *Biol. Reprod.* **15,** 555–560.

Erickson, G. F. and Hsueh, A. J. W. (1978). Stimulation of aromatase activity by follicle stimulating hormone in rat granulosa cells *in vivo* and *in vitro*. *Endocrinology* **102,** 1275–1282.

Erickson, G. F., Hsueh, A. J. W., Quigley, M. E., Rebar, R. W. and Yen, S. S. C. (1979). Functional studies of aromatase activity in human granulosa cells from normal and polycystic ovaries. *J. Clin. Endocrinol. Metab.* **49,** 514–519.

Erickson, J. D. (1978). Down syndrome, paternal age, maternal age and birth order. *Ann. Hum. Genet.* **41,** 289–298.

Ernster, V. L. and Petrakis, N. L. (1981). Effect of hormonal events in earlier life and socioeconomic status on age at menopause. *Am. J. Obstet. Gynecol.* **140,** 471–472.

Eshkol, A., Lunenfeld, B. and Peters, H. (1971). Ovarian development in infant mice. *In* "Gonadotrophins and Ovarian Development" (W. R. Butt, A. C. Crooke and M. Ryle, eds.), pp. 249–258. Livingstone, Edinburgh.

Evans, J. A., Hunter, A. G. W. and Hamerton, J. L. (1978). Down syndrome and recent demographic trends in Manitoba. *J. Med. Genet.* **15,** 43–47.

Everett, J. W. (1939). Spontaneous persistent estrus in a strain of albino rats. *Endocrinology* **25,** 123–127.

Everett, J. W. (1940). The restoration of ovulatory cycles and corpus luteum formation in persistent-estrous rats by progesterone. *Endocrinology* **27,** 681–686.

Everett, J. W. (1970). Photoregulation of the ovarian cycle in the rat. *In* "La photorégulation de la reproduction chez les oiseaux et les mammifères" (J. Benoit and I. Assenmacher, eds.), pp. 387–403. CNRS, Paris.

Everett, J. W. (1974). A neural timepiece for ovulation? *Anat. Rec.* **180,** 151–156.

Everett, J. W. (1980). Reinstatement of estrous cycles in middle-aged spontaneously persistent estrous rats: Importance of circulating prolactin and the resulting facilitative action of progesterone. *Endocrinology* **106**, 1691–1696.

Everett, J. W. and Sawyer, C. H. (1950). A 24-hour periodicity in the "LH-release apparatus" of female rats, disclosed by barbiturate sedation. *Endocrinology* **47**, 198–218.

Everett, J. W. and Tyrey, L. (1983). Comparable surges of luteinizing hormone induced by preoptic or medial basal tuberal electrical stimulation in spontaneously persistent estrous or cyclic proestrous rats. *Endocrinology* **112**, 2015–2020.

Fabricant, J. D., Dunn, G. and Schneider, E. L. (1978). Maternal age-related pre- and postimplantation fetal mortality: A strain survey. *Mech. Ageing Dev.* **8**, 227–231.

Faddy, M. J., Jones, E. C. and Edwards, R. G. (1976). An analytical model for ovarian follicle dynamics. *J. Exp. Zool.* **197**, 173–186.

Faddy, M. J., Gosden, R. G. and Edwards, R. G. (1983). Ovarian follicle dynamics in mice: A comparative study of three inbred strains and an F1 hybrid. *J. Endocrinol.* **96**, 23–33.

Falck, B. (1959). Site of production of oestrogen in rat ovary as studied in micro-transplants. *Acta Physiol., Scand.* **47**, Suppl. 163, 1–101.

Farish, E., Fletcher, C. D., Hart, D. M., Azzawi, F. A., Abdalla, H. I. and Gray, C. E. (1984). The effects of hormone implants on serum lipoproteins and steroid hormones in bilaterally ovariectomized women. *Acta Endocrinol. Copenhagen* **106**, 116–120.

Farley, J. R., Wergedal, J. E. and Baylink, D. J. (1983). Fluoride directly stimulates proliferation and alkaline phosphatase activity of bone-forming cells. *Science* **222**, 330–332.

Fédération CECOS, Schwartz, D. and Mayaux, M. J. (1982). Female fecundity as a function of age. Results of artificial insemination in 2193 nulliparous women with azoospermic husbands. *N. Engl. J. Med.* **306**, 404–406.

Felicio, L. S., Nelson, J. F. and Finch, C. E. (1980). Spontaneous pituitary tumorigenesis and plasma oestradiol in ageing female C57BL/6J mice. *Exp. Gerontol.* **15**, 139–143.

Felicio, L. S., Nelson, J. F., Gosden, R. G. and Finch, C. E. (1983). Restoration of ovulatory cycles by ovarian grafts in aging mice: Potentiation by long-term ovariectomy decreases with age. *Proc. Natl. Acad. Sci. U.S.A.* **80**, 6076–6080.

Felicio, L. S., Finch, C. E., Gosden, R. G. and Nelson, J. F. (1984). Effects of long-term ovariectomy on the potential for oestrous cyclicity and pregnancy disclosed by ovarian grafts in ageing mice. *J. Physiol. (London)* **346**, 122P.

Fergusson, I. L. C., Taylor, R. W. and Watson, J. M. (1982). "Records and Curiosities in Obstetrics and Gynaecology." Baillière, London.

Ferin, M., Antunes, J. L., Zimmerman, E., Dyrenfurth, I., Frantz, A. G., Robinson, A. and Carmel, P. W. (1977). Endocrine function in female rhesus monkeys after hypothalamic disconnection. *Endocrinology* **101**, 1611–1620.

Fienberg, R. (1969). The stromal theca cell and postmenopausal endometrial adenocarcinoma. *Cancer* **24**, 32–38.

Finch, C. E. (1976). The regulation of physiological changes during mammalian aging. *Q. Rev. Biol.* **51**, 49–83.

Finch, C. E., Felicio, L. S., Flurkey, K., Gee, D. M., Mobbs, C., Nelson, J. F. and Osterburg, H. H. (1980). Studies on ovarian-hypothalamic-pituitary interactions during reproductive aging in C57BL/6J mice. *Peptides* **1**, Suppl. 1, 163–175.

Finch, C. E., Marshall, J. F. and Randall, P. K. (1981). Aging and basal ganglion functions. *Annu. Rev. Gerontol. Geriatr.* **2**, 49–87.

Finn, C. A. (1964). Influence of the male on litter size in mice. *J. Reprod. Fertil.* **7**, 107–111.

Finn, C. A. (1966). The initiation of the decidual cell reaction in the uterus of the aged mouse. *J. Reprod. Fertil.* **11**, 423–428.

Finn, C. A. (1970). The ageing uterus and its influence on reproductive capacity. *J. Reprod. Fertil. Suppl.* **12**, 31–38.

Finn, C. A. and Martin, L. (1970). The role of the oestrogen secreted before oestrus in the preparation of the uterus for implantation in the mouse. *J. Endocrinol.* **47**, 431–438.

Finney, D. J. (1971). "Probit Analysis," 3rd ed. Cambridge Univ. Press, London and New York.

Fishman, J. (1981). Biological action of catechol oestrogens. *J. Endocrinol.* **89**, 59P–65P.

Fishman, J. and Norton, B. (1975). Catechol estrogen formation in the central nervous system of the rat. *Endocrinology* **96**, 1054–1059.

Fishman, J., Boyar, R. M. and Hellman, L. (1975). Influence of body weight on estradiol metabolism in young women. *J. Clin. Endocrinol. Metab.* **41**, 989–991.

Flickinger, G. L., Elsner, C., Illingworth, D. V., Muechler, E. K. and Mikhail, G. (1977). Estrogen and progesterone receptors in the female genital tract of humans and monkeys. *Ann. N.Y. Acad. Sci.* **286**, 180–189.

Flint, M. (1976). Cross-cultural factors that affect age of menopause. *In* "Consensus on Menopause Research" (P. A. van Keep, R. B. Greenblatt and M. Albeaux-Fernet, eds.), pp. 73–83. MTP Press, Lancaster.

Flint, M. P. and Garcia, M. (1979). Culture and the climacteric. *J. Biosocial Sci., Suppl.* **6**, 197–215.

Flurkey, K., Gee, D. M., Sinha, Y. N., Wisner, J. R., Jr. and Finch, C. E. (1982). Age effects on luteinizing hormone, progesterone and prolactin in proestrous and acyclic C57BL/6J mice. *Biol. Reprod.* **26**, 835–846.

Fortune, J. E. and Armstrong, D. T. (1977). Androgen production by theca and granulosa isolated from proestrous rat follicles. *Endocrinology* **100**, 1341–1347.

Fothergill, J. (1776). On the management proper at the cessation of the menses. *Med. Observ. Enquiries* **5**, 160–186; reprinted in "Essays on the Puerperal Fever and other Diseases Peculiar to Women. Selected from the Writings of British Authors Previous to the Close of the Eighteenth Century" (F. Churchill, ed.), pp. 503–516. Sydenham Soc. Publ., London, 1849.

Francis, R. M., Peacock, M., Taylor, G. A., Storer, J. H. and Nordin, B. E. C. (1984). Calcium malabsorption in elderly women with vertebral fractures: Evidence for resistance to the action of vitamin D metabolites on the bowel. *Clin. Sci.* **66**, 103–107.

Fraser, H. M., McNeilly, A. S. and Popkin, R. M. (1984). Passive immunization against LHRH: elucidation of the role of LHRH in controlling LH and FSH secretion and LHRH receptors. *In* "Immunological Aspects of Reproduction in Mammals" (B. G. Crighton, ed.), pp. 399–418. Butterworth, London (in press).

Frazer, J. G. (1935). "The Golden Bough. A Study in Magic and Religion." Macmillan, New York.

Frere, G. (1971). Mean age at menopause and menarche in South Africa. *S. Afr. J. Med. Sci.* **36**, 21–24.

Friedrich, F., Kemeter, P., Salzer, H. and Breitenecker, G. (1975). Ovulation inhibition with human chorionic gonadotrophin. *Acta Endocrinol. (Copenhagen)* **78**, 332–342.

Frisch, R. E., Canick, J. A. and Tulchinsky, D. (1980). Human fatty marrow aromatizes androgen to estrogen. *J. Clin. Endocrinol. Metab.* **51**, 394–396.

Frommer, D. J. (1964). Changing age of menopause. *Br. Med. J.* **2**, 349–351.

Frumar, A. M., Meldrum, D. R., Geola, F., Shamonki, I. M., Tataryn, I. V., Deftos, L. J. and Judd, H. L. (1980). Relationship of fasting urinary calcium to circulating estrogen and body weight in post-menopausal women. *J. Clin. Endocrinol. Metab.* **50**, 70–75.

Fugo, N. W. and Butcher, R. L. (1971). Effects of prolonged estrous cycles on reproduction in aged rats. *Fertil. Steril.* **22**, 98–101.

Gaddum-Rosse, P., Rumery, R. E., Blandau, R. J. and Thiersch, J. B. (1975). Studies on the mucosa of postmenopausal oviducts: Surface appearance, ciliary activity, and the effect of estrogen treatment. *Fertil. Steril.* **26**, 951–969.

Gallagher, J. C., Young, M. M. and Nordin, B. E. C. (1972). Effects of artificial menopause on plasma and urine calcium and phosphate. *Clin. Endocrinol. (Oxford)* **1**, 57–64.

Gallagher, J. C., Riggs, B. L., Eisman, J., Hamstra, A., Arnaud, S. B. and DeLuca, H. F. (1979). Intestinal calcium absorption and serum vitamin D metabolites in normal subjects and os-teoporotic patients. *J. Clin. Invest.* **64**, 729–736.

Gallagher, J. C., Melton, L. J., Riggs, B. L. and Bergstrath, E. (1980a). Epidemiology of fractures of the proximal femur in Rochester, Minnesota. *Clin. Orthop.* **150**, 163–171.

Gallagher, J. C., Riggs, B. L. and DeLuca, H. F. (1980b). Effect of estrogen on calcium absorption and serum vitamin D metabolites in postmenopausal osteoporosis. *J. Clin. Endocrinol. Metab.* **51**, 1359–1364.

Gallagher, J. C., Jerpbak, C. M., Jee, W. S. S., Johnson, K. A., DeLuca, H. F. and Riggs, B. L. (1982). 1,25-dihydroxyvitamin D3: short- and long-term effects on bone and calcium metabo-lism in patients with postmenopausal osteoporosis. *Proc. Natl. Acad. Sci. U.S.A.* **79**, 3325–3329.

Gallo, R. V. and Kalra, P. S. (1983). Pulsatile LH release on diestrus I in the rat estrous cycle: Relation to brain catecholamines and ovarian steroid secretion. *Neuroendocrinology* **37**, 91–97.

Gambrell, R. D., Jr., Massey, F. M., Castaneda, T. A., Ugenas, A. J., Ricci, C. A. and Wright, J. M. (1980). Use of the progestogen challenge test to reduce the risk of endometrial cancer. *Obstet. Gynecol.* **55**, 732–738.

Gardner, R. L. and Rossant, J. (1976). Determination during embryogenesis. *Ciba Found. Symp.* [N.S] **40**, 5–25.

Garfinkel, J. and Selvin, S. (1976). A multivariate analysis of the relationship between parental age and birth order and the human secondary sex ratio. *J. Biosocial Sci.* **8**, 113–121.

Gartler, S. M., Liskay, R. M. and Gant, N. (1973). Two functional X chromosomes in human fetal oocytes. *Exp. Cell Res.* **82**, 464–466.

Gee, D. M., Flurkey, K. and Finch, C. E. (1983). Aging and the regulation of luteinizing hormone in C57BL/6J mice: Impaired elevations after ovariectomy and spontaneous elevations at ad-vanced ages. *Biol. Reprod.* **28**, 598–607.

German, J. (1968). Mongolism, delayed fertilization and human sexual behaviour. *Nature (London)* **217**, 516–518.

German, J., Simpson, S. L., Chaganti, R. S. K., Summitt, R. L., Reid, L. B. and Merkatz, I. R. (1978). Genetically determined sex-reversal in 46,XY humans. *Science* **202**, 53–56.

Gesell, M. S. and Roth, G. S. (1981). Decrease in rat uterine estrogen receptors during aging: Physio- and immunochemical properties. *Endocrinology* **109**, 1502–1508.

Ginsburg, J. and O'Reilly, B. (1983). Climacteric flushing in a man. *Br. Med. J.* **287**, 262.

Ginsburg, J., Swinhoe, J. and O'Reilly, B. (1981). Cardiovascular responses during the menopausal hot flush. *Br. J. Obstet. Gynaecol.* **88**, 925–930.

Giorgi, E. P. (1963). The determination of steroids in cyst fluid from human polycystic ovaries. *J. Endocrinol.* **27**, 225–240.

Golbus, M. S. (1983). Oocyte sensitivity to induced meiotic non-disjunction and its relationship to advanced maternal age. *Am. J. Obstet. Gynecol.* **146**, 435–438.

Goldenberg, R. L., Grodin, J. M., Rodbard, D. and Ross, G. T. (1973). Gonadotropins in women with amenorrhea. The use of plasma follicle-stimulating hormone to differentiate women with and without ovarian follicles. *Am. J. Obstet. Gynecol.* **116**, 1003–1012.

Goldin, B. R. and Gorbach, S. L. (1976). The relationship between diet and rat fecal bacterial enzymes implicated in colon cancer. *J. Natl. Cancer Inst. (U.S.)* **57**, 371–375.

Goldin, B. R., Aldercreutz, H., Dwyer, J. T., Swenson, L., Warram, J. H. and Gorbach, S. L. (1981). Effect of diet on excretion of estrogens in pre- and postmenopausal women. *Cancer Res.* **41**, 3771–3773.

Goldman, R. (1977). Ageing of the excretory system: Kidney and bladder. *In* ''Handbook of the Biology of Aging'' (C. E. Finch and L. Hayflick, eds.), pp. 409–431. Van Nostrand-Reinhold, Princeton, New Jersey.

Goldsmith, O., Solomon, D. H. and Horton, R. (1967). Hypogonadism and mineralocorticoid excess. The 17-hydroxylase deficiency syndrome. *N. Engl. J. Med.* **277**, 673–677.

Goodlin, R. C. (1965). Nondisjunction and maternal age in the mouse. *J. Reprod. Fertil.* **9**, 355–356.

Goodman, A. L. and Hodgen, G. D. (1979). Between-ovary interactions in the regulation of follicle growth, corpus luteum function, and gonadotropin secretion in the primate ovarian cycle. II. Effects of luteectomy and hemiovariectomy during the luteal phase in cynomolgus monkeys. *Endocrinology* **104**, 1310–1316.

Goodman, A. L., Nixon, W. E., Johnson, D. K. and Hodgen, G. D. (1977). Regulation of folliculogenesis in the cycling rhesus monkey: Selection of the dominant follicle. *Endocrinology* **100**, 155–161.

Goodman, R. L. (1978). The site of positive feedback action of estradiol in the rat. *Endocrinology* **102**, 151–159.

Gordon, T., Castelli, W. P., Hjortland, M. C., Kannel, W. B. and Dawber, T. R. (1977). High density lipoprotein as a protective factor against coronary heart disease: The Framingham Study. *Am. J. Med.* **62**, 707–714.

Gordon, T., Kannel, W. B., Hjortland, M. C. and McNamara, P. M. (1978). Menopause and coronary heart disease. The Framingham Study. *Ann. Intern. Med.* **89**, 157–161.

Gosden, R. G. (1979). Effects of age and parity on the breeding performance of mice with one or two ovaries. *J. Reprod. Fertil.* **57**, 477–487.

Gosden, R. G. and Fowler, R. E. (1979). Corpus luteum function in ageing inbred mice. *Experientia* **35**, 128–129.

Gosden, R. G. and Russell, J. A. (1981). Spontaneous abdominal implantation in the rat with development to full term. *Lab. Anim.* **15**, 379–380.

Gosden, R. G., Hawkins, H. K. and Gosden, C. A. (1978). Autofluorescent particles of human uterine muscle cells. *Am. J. Pathol.* **91**, 155–174.

Gosden, R. G., Holinka, C. F. and Finch, C. E. (1981). The distribution of fetal mortality in ageing C57BL/6J mice: A statistical analysis. *Exp. Gerontol.* **16**, 127–130.

Gosden, R. G., Laing, S. C., Felicio, L. S., Nelson, J. F. and Finch, C. E. (1983a). Imminent oocyte exhaustion and reduced follicular recruitment mark the transition to acyclicity in aging C57BL/6J mice. *Biol. Reprod.* **28**, 255–260.

Gosden, R. G., Laing, S. C., Flurkey, K. and Finch, C. E. (1983b). Graafian follicle growth and replacement in anovulatory ovaries of ageing C57BL/6J mice. *J. Reprod. Fertil.* **69**, 453–462.

Gougeon, A. (1982). Rate of follicular growth in the human ovary. *In* ''Follicular Maturation and Ovulation'' (R. Rolland, E. V. van Hall, S. G. Hillier, K. P. McNatty and J. Schoemaker, eds.), pp. 155–163. Excerpta Medica, Amsterdam.

Gougeon, A. and Lefévre, B. (1983). Evolution of the diameters of the largest healthy and atretic follicles during the human menstrual cycle. *J. Reprod. Fertil.* **69**, 497–502.

Gould, K. G., Flint, M. and Graham, C. E. (1981). Chimpanzee reproductive senescence: A possible model for evolution of the menopause. *Maturitas* **3**, 157–166.

Graham, C. E. (1979). Reproductive function in aged female chimpanzees. *Am. J. Phys. Anthropol.* **50**, 291–300.

Graham, C. E., Kling, O. R. and Steiner, R. A. (1979). Reproductive senescence in female nonhuman primates. *In* ''Aging in Non-human Primates'' (D. M. Bowden, ed.), pp. 183–202. Van Nostrand-Reinhold, Princeton, New Jersey.

Gray, R. H. (1976). The menopause - epidemiological and demographic considerations. *In* ''The

Menopause: A Guide to Current Research and Practice'' (R. J. Beard, ed.), pp. 25–40. MTP Press, Lancaster.

Gray, R. H. (1979). Biological and social interactions in the determination of late fertility. *J. Biosocial Sci. Suppl.* **6**, 97–115.

Greenblatt, R. B., Colle, M. L. and Mahesh, V. B. (1976). Ovarian and adrenal steroid production in the postmenopausal woman. *Obstet. Gynecol.* **47**, 383–387.

Greenblatt, R. B., Nezhat, C. and McNamara, V. P. (1979). Appropriate contraception for middle-aged women. *J. Biosocial Sci., Suppl.* **6**, 119–141.

Grodin, J. M., Siiteri, P. K. and MacDonald, P. C. (1973). Source of estrogen production in postmenopausal women. *J. Clin. Endocrinol. Metab.* **36**, 207–214.

Gropp, A. (1976). Morphological consequences of trisomy in mammals. *Ciba Found. Symp.* [N.S.] **40**, 155–171.

Guttmacher, A. F. (1956). Factors affecting normal expectancy of conception. *JAMA, J. Am. Med. Assoc.* **161**, 855–860.

Hafez, E. S. E. (1982). Scanning electron microscopy of female reproductive organs during meno-pause and related pathologies. *In* ''The Menopause: Clinical, Endocrinological and Pathophys-iological Aspects'' (P. Fioretti, L. Martini, G. B. Melis and S. S. C. Yen, eds.), Serono Found. Symp. No. 39, pp. 201–217. Academic Press, New York.

Hagen, C., Christensen, M. S., Christiansen, C., Stocklund, K.-E., and Transbøl, I. (1982a). Effects of two years' estrogen-gestagen replacement on climacteric symptoms and gonadotropins in the early postmenopausal period. *Acta Obstet. Gynecol. Scand.* **61**, 237–241.

Hagen, C., Christiansen, C., Christensen, M. S. and Transbøl, I. (1982b). Climacteric symptoms, fat mass, and plasma concentrations of LH, FSH, Prl, oestradiol-17β and androstenedione in the early post-menopausal period. *Acta Endocrinol. (Copenhagen)* **101**, 87–92.

Hallström, T. (1979). Sexuality of women in middle age: The Göteborg study. *J. Biosocial Sci., Suppl.* **6**, 165–175.

Hammond, C. B. and Maxson, W. S. (1982). Current status of estrogen therapy for the menopause. *Fertil. Steril.* **37**, 5–25.

Hammond, C. B., Jelovsek, F. R., Lee, K. L., Creasman, W. T. and Parker, R. T. (1979a). Effects of long-term estrogen replacement therapy. I. Metabolic effects. *Am. J. Obstet. Gynecol.* **133**, 525–536.

Hammond, C. B., Jelovsek, F. R., Lee, K. L., Creasman, W. T. and Parker, R. T. (1979b). Effects of long-term estrogen replacement therapy. II. Neoplasia. *Am. J. Obstet. Gynecol.* **133**, 537–547.

Harris, G. W. (1972). Humours and hormones. *J. Endocrinol.* **53**, ii–xxiii.

Harrison, J. E., McNeill, K. G., Sturtridge, W. C., Bayley, T. A., Murray, T. M., Williams, C., Tam, C. and Fornasier, V. (1981). Three-year changes in bone mineral mass of postmeno-pausal osteoporotic patients based on neutron activation analysis of the central third of the skeleton. *J. Clin. Endocrinol. Metab.* **52**, 751–758.

Hasselquist, M. B., Goldberg, N., Schroeter, A. and Spelsberg, T. C. (1980). Isolation and charac-terization of the estrogen receptor in human skin. *J. Clin. Endocrinol. Metab.* **50**, 76–82.

Hassold, T., Jacobs, P., Kline, J., Stein, Z. and Warburton, D. (1980). Effect of maternal age on autosomal trisomies. *Ann. Hum. Genet.* **44**, 29–36.

Hauser, G. A., Obiri, J. A., Valaer, M., Erb, H., Müeller, T., Remen, U. and Vanäänen, P. (1961). Der Einfluss des Menarchealters auf des Menopausealter. *Gynaecologia* **152**, 279–286.

Hauser, G. A., Remen, U., Valaer, M., Erb, H., Müeller, T. and Obiri, J. (1963). Menarche and menopause in Israel. *Gynaecologia* **155**, 38–47.

Hay, M. F., Moor, R. M., Cran, D. G. and Dott, H. M. (1979). Regeneration of atretic ovarian follicles *in vitro*. *J. Reprod. Fertil.* **55**, 195–207.

Heaney, R. P., Recker, R. R. and Saville, P. D. (1978a). Menopausal changes in calcium balance performance. *J. Lab. Clin. Med.* **92**, 953–963.

Heaney, R. P., Recker, R. R. and Saville, P. D. (1978b). Menopausal changes in bone remodelling. *J. Lab. Clin. Med.* **92**, 964–970.

Hegner, R. W. (1914). "The Germ Cell Cycle in Animals." Macmillan, New York.

Henderson, S. A. and Edwards, R. G. (1968). Chiasma frequency and maternal age in mammals. *Nature (London)* **218**, 22–28.

Hendricks, S. E., Lehman, J. R. and Oswalt, G. L. (1979). Effects of copulation on reproductive function in aged female rats. *Physiol. Behav.* **23**, 267–272.

Henneman, D. (1968). Effect of estrogen on *in vivo* and *in vitro* collagen biosynthesis and maturation in old and young female guinea pigs. *Endocrinology* **83**, 678–690.

Henry, L. (1961). Some data on natural fertility. *Eugen. Q.* **8**, 81–91.

Hermann, W. J., Jr. (1982). The effect of vitamin E on lipoprotein cholesterol distribution. *Ann. N.Y. Acad. Sci.* **393**, 467–471.

Hertig, A. T. (1967). The overall problem in man. *In* "Comparative Aspects of Reproductive Failure" (K. Benirschke, ed.), pp. 11–41. Springer-Verlag, Berlin and New York.

Hertig, A. T., Rock, J., Adams, E. C. and Menkin, M. C. (1959). Thirty-four fertilized human ova, good, bad and indifferent, recovered from 210 women of known fertility. *Pediatrics* **23**, 202–211.

Hill, P., Garbaczewski, L., Helman, P., Huskisson, J., Sporangisa, E. and Wynder, E. L. (1980). Diet, lifestyle and menstrual activity. *Am. J. Clin. Nutr.* **33**, 1192–1198.

Hillier, S. G. and de Zwart, F. A. (1981). Evidence that granulosa cell aromatase induction/activation by follicle-stimulating hormone is an androgen receptor-regulated process *in vitro*. *Endocrinology* **109**, 1303–1305.

Hillier, S. G., Reichert, L. E., Jr. and van Hall, E. V. (1981). Control of preovulatory follicular estrogen biosynthesis in the human ovary. *J. Clin. Endocrinol. Metab.* **52**, 847–856.

Himelstein-Braw, R., Peters, H. and Faber, M. (1977). Influence of irradiation and chemotherapy on the ovaries of children with abdominal tumours. *Br. J. Cancer* **36**, 269–275.

Himelstein-Braw, R., Peters, H. and Faber, M. (1978). Morphological study of the ovaries of leukaemic children. *Br. J. Cancer* **38**, 82–87.

Hirshfield, A. N. and Midgley, A. R., Jr. (1978). The role of FSH in the selection of large ovarian follicles in the rat. *Biol. Reprod.* **19**, 606–611.

Hjortland, M. C., McNamara, P. M. and Kannel, W. B. (1976). Some atherogenic concomitants of menopause: the Framingham Study. *Am. J. Epidemiol.* **103**, 304–311.

Hoak, D. C., and Schwartz, N. B. (1980). Blockade of recruitment of ovarian follicles by suppression of the secondary surge of follicle-stimulating hormone with porcine follicular fluid. *Proc. Natl. Acad. Sci. U.S.A.* **77**, 4953–4956.

Hodgen, G. D., Goodman, A. L., O'Connor, A. and Johnson, D. K. (1977). Menopause in rhesus monkeys: Model for study of disorders of the human climacteric. *Am. J. Obstet. Gynecol.* **127**, 581–584.

Hofmann, D. and Soergel, T. (1972). Studies on the age of menarche and the age of menopause. *Geburtshilfe Frauenheilkd.* **32**, 969–977.

Hohlweg, W. and Junkmann, K. (1932). Die hormonal-nervöse Regulierung der Funktion des Hypophysenvorderlappens. *Klin. Wochenschr.* **11**, 321–323.

Højager, B., Peters, H., Byskov, A. G. and Faber, M. (1978). Follicular development in ovaries of children with Down's syndrome. *Acta Paediatr. Scand.* **67**, 637–643.

Holinka, C. F. and Finch, C. E. (1977). Age-related changes in the decidual response of the C57BL/6J mouse uterus. *Biol. Reprod.* **16**, 385–393.

Holinka, C. F., Hetland, M. D. and Finch, C. E. (1977). The response to a single dose of estradiol in the uterus of ovariectomized C57BL/6J mice during aging. *Biol. Reprod.* **17**, 262–264.

Holinka, C. F., Tseng, Y.-C. and Finch, C. E. (1978). Prolonged gestation, elevated preparuritional plasma progesterone and reproductive aging in C57BL/6J mice. *Biol. Reprod.* **19**, 807–816.

Holinka, C. F., Tseng, Y.-C. and Finch, C. E. (1979). Reproductive aging in C57BL/6J mice: plasma progesterone, viable embryos and resorption frequency throughout pregnancy. *Biol. Reprod.* **20**, 1201–1211.

Honoré, L. H., Dill, F. J. and Poland, B. J. (1976). Placental morphology in spontaneous human abortuses with normal and abnormal karyotypes. *Teratology* **14**, 151–166.

Hook, E. B. (1981). Rates of chromosome abnormalities at different maternal ages. *Obstet. Gynecol. (N.Y.)* **58**, 282–285.

Hook, E. B. (1983). Down syndrome rates and relaxed selection at older maternal ages. *Am. J. Hum. Genet.* **35**, 1307–1313.

Horsman, A., Jones, M., Francis, R. and Nordin, C. (1983). The effect of estrogen dose on postmenopausal bone loss. *N. Engl. J. Med.* **309**, 1405–1407.

Horton, R. and Tait, J. F. (1966). Androstenedione production and interconversion rates measured in peripheral blood and studies on the possible site of its conversion to testosterone. *J. Clin. Invest.* **45**, 301–313.

Horton, R. and Tait, J. F. (1967). *In vivo* conversion of dehydroisoandrosterone to plasma androstenedione and testosterone in man. *J. Clin. Endocrinol. Metab.* **27**, 79–88.

Howard, G., Blair, M., Fotherby, K., Trayner, I., Hamauri, A. and Elder, M. G. (1982). Some metabolic effects of long-term use of the injectable contraceptive norethisterone oenanthate. *Lancet* **1**, 423–425.

Huang, H. H. and Meites, J. (1975). Reproductive capacity of aging female rats. *Neuroendocrinology* **17**, 289–295.

Huang, H. H., Marshall, S. and Meites, J. (1976). Induction of estrous cycles in old non-cyclic rats by progesterone, ACTH, ether stress or L-DOPA. *Neuroendocrinology* **20**, 21–34.

Hunter, D. J. S., Anderson, A. B. M. and Haddon, M. (1979). Changes in coagulation factors in postmenopausal women on ethinyl oestradiol. *Br. J. Obstet. Gynaecol.* **86**, 488–490.

Hunter, J. (1787). An experiment to determine the effect of extirpating one ovarium upon the number of young produced. *Philos. Trans. R. Soc. London, Ser. B* **77**, 233–239.

Ingram, D. L., Mandl, A. M. and Zuckerman, S. (1958). The influence of age on litter size. *J. Endocrinol.* **17**, 280–285.

Insogna, K. L., Lewis, A. M., Lipinski, B. A., Bryant, C. and Baran, D. T. (1981). Effect of age on serum immunoreactive parathyroid hormone and its biological effects. *J. Clin. Endocrinol. Metab.* **53**, 1072–1075.

Ireland, P. and Fordtran, J. S. (1973). Effect of dietary calcium and age on jejunal calcium absorption in humans studied by intestinal perfusion. *J. Clin. Invest.* **52**, 2672–2681.

Iskrant, A. P. (1968). The etiology of fractured hips in females. *Am. J. Public Health* **58**, 485–490.

Israel, S. L. and Deutschberger, J. (1964). Relation of the mothers' age to obstetric performance. *Obstet. Gynecol. (N.Y.)* **24**, 411–417.

Jacobs, P. A. and Hassold, T. J. (1980). The origin of chromosome abnormalities in spontaneous abortions. *In* "Human Embryonic and Fetal Death" (I. H. Porter and E. B. Hook, eds.), pp. 289–298. Academic Press, New York.

Jacobs, P. A., Angell, R. R., Buchanan, I. M., Hassold, T. J., Matsuyama, A. M. and Manuel, B. (1978). The origin of human triploids. *Ann. Hum. Genet.* **42**, 49–57.

James, W. H. (1974a). Spontaneous abortion and birth order. *J. Biosocial Sci.* **6**, 23–41.

James, W. H. (1974b). Marital coital rates, spouses' ages, family size and social class. *J. Sex Res.* **10**, 205–218.

James, W. H. (1979). Maternal age, dizygotic twinning rates and age at menopause. *Ann. Hum. Biol.* **6**, 481–483.

Jaszmann, L., van Lith, N. D. and Zaat, J. C. A. (1969a). The perimenopausal symptoms: The statistical analysis of a survey. *Med. Gynaecol. Sociol.* **4**, 268–277.

Jaszmann, L., van Lith, N. D. and Zaat, J. C. A. (1969b). The age at menopause in the Netherlands. *Int. J. Fertil.* **14**, 106–117.

Jick, H., Porter, J. and Morrison, A. S. (1977). Relation between smoking and age of natural menopause. *Lancet* **1**, 1354–1355.

Jick, H., Dinan, B. and Rothman, K. J. (1978a). Oral contraceptives and non-fatal myocardial infarction. *JAMA, J. Am. Med. Assoc.* **239**, 1403–1406.

Jick, H., Dinan, B. and Rothman, K. J. (1978b). Non-contraceptive oestrogens and non-fatal myocardial infarction. *JAMA, J. Am. Med. Assoc.* **239**, 1407–1408.

Johansson, E. D. B. (1969). Progesterone levels in peripheral plasma during the luteal phase of the normal human menstrual cycle measured by a rapid competitive protein binding technique. *Acta Endocrinol. (Copenhagen)* **61**, 592–606.

Jones, E. C. (1970). The ageing ovary and its influence on reproductive capacity. *J. Reprod. Fertil., Suppl.* **12**, 17–30.

Jones, E. C. and Krohn, P. L. (1959). Influence of the anterior pituitary on the ageing process in the ovary. *Nature (London)* **183**, 1155–1158.

Jones, E. C. and Krohn, P. L. (1960). The effect of unilateral ovariectomy on the reproductive lifespan of mice. *J. Endocrinol.* **20**, 129–134.

Jones, E. C. and Krohn, P. L. (1961a). The relationships between age, numbers of oocytes and fertility in virgin and multiparous mice. *J. Endocrinol.* **21**, 469–495.

Jones, E. C. and Krohn, P. L. (1961b). The effect of hypophysectomy on age changes in the ovaries of mice. *J. Endocrinol.* **21**, 497–508.

Jones, G. S. and de Moraes-Ruehsen, M. (1969). A new syndrome of amenorrhea in association with hypergonadotropism and apparently normal ovarian follicular apparatus. *Am. J. Obstet. Gynecol.* **104**, 597–600.

Jongbloet, P. H. (1975). The effects of preovulatory overripeness of human eggs on development. *In* "Aging Gametes" (R. J. Blandau, ed.), pp. 300–329. Karger, Basel.

Judd, H. L. and Korenman, S. G. (1982). Effects of aging on reproductive function in women. *In* "Endocrine Aspects of Aging" (S. G. Korenman, ed.), pp. 163–197. Am. Elsevier, New York.

Judd, H. L. and Yen, S. S. C. (1973). Serum androstenedione and testosterone levels during the menstrual cycle. *J. Clin. Endocrinol. Metab.* **36**, 475–481.

Judd, H. L., Judd, G. E., Lucas, W. E. and Yen, S. S. C. (1974a). Endocrine function of the postmenopausal ovary: Concentration of androgens and estrogens in ovarian and peripheral vein blood. *J. Clin. Endocrinol. Metab.* **39**, 1020–1024.

Judd, H. L., Lucas, W. E. and Yen, S. S. C. (1974b). Effect of oophorectomy on circulating testosterone and androstenedione levels in patients with endometrial cancer. *Am. J. Obstet. Gynecol.* **118**, 793–798.

Judd, H. L., Shamonki, I. M., Frumar, A. M. and Lagasse, L. D. (1982). Origin of serum estradiol in postmenopausal women. *Obstet. Gynecol. (N.Y.)* **59**, 680–686.

Kao, K. Y. T., Hitt, W. E. and Leslie, J. G. (1976). The intermolecular cross-links in uterine collagens of guinea pig, pig, cow and human beings. *Proc. Soc. Exp. Biol. Med.* **151**, 385–389.

Kaufman, D. W., Slone, D., Rosenberg, L., Miettinen, O. S. and Shapiro, S. (1980). Cigarette smoking and age at natural menopause. *Am. J. Public Health* **70**, 420–422.

Kaufman, F. R., Kogut, M. D., Donnell, G. N., Goebelsmann, U., March, C. and Koch, R. (1981). Hypergonadotropic hypogonadism in female patients with galactosemia. *New Engl. J. Med.* **304**, 994–998.

Kennedy, N. S. J., Eastell, R., Ferrington, C. M., Simpson, J. D., Smith, M. A., Strong, J. A. and Tothill, P. (1982). Total body neutron activation analysis of calcium: Calibration and normalisation. *Phys. Med. Biol.* **27**, 697–707.

Kennedy, T. G. (1977). Evidence for a role of prostaglandins in the initiation of blastocyst implantation in the rat. *Biol. Reprod.* **16**, 286–291.

Kennedy, T. G. and Kennedy, J. P. (1972). Effects of age and parity on reproduction in young female mice. *J. Reprod. Fertil.* **28**, 77–84.

King, C. R., Magenis, E. and Bennett, S. (1978). Pregnancy and the Turner syndrome. *Obstet. Gynecol. (N.Y.)* **52**, 617–624.

Kinsey, A. C., Pomeroy, W. B., Martin, C. E. and Gebhard, P. H. (1953). "Sexual Behaviour in the Human Female." Saunders, Philadelphia, Pennsylvania.

Kitabchi, A. E. (1980). Hormonal status in vitamin E deficiency. *Basic Clin. Nutr.* **1**, 348–371.

Kline, J., Levin, B., Shrout, P., Stein, Z., Susser, M. and Warburton, D. (1983). Maternal smoking and trisomy among spontaneously aborted conceptions. *Am. J. Hum. Genet.* **35**, 421–431.

Knauer, E. (1896). II. Einige Versuche über Ovarientransplantation bei Kaninchen. *Zentralbl. Gynaekol.* **20**, 524–528.

Knobil, E. (1974). On the control of gonadotropin secretion in the rhesus monkey. *Recent Prog. Horm. Res.* **30**, 1–36.

Knobil, E., Plant, T. M., Wildt, L., Belchetz, P. E. and Marshall, G. (1980). Control of the rhesus monkey menstrual cycle: Permissive role of hypothalamic gonadotropin-releasing hormone. *Science* **207**, 1371–1373.

Kohler, P. O., Ross, G. T. and Odell, W. D. (1968). Metabolic clearance and production rates of human luteinizing hormone in pre- and postmenopausal women. *J. Clin. Invest.* **47**, 38–47.

Korenman, S. G., Perrin, L. E. and McCallam, T. P. (1969). A radio-ligand binding assay system for estradiol measurement in human plasma. *J. Clin. Endocrinol. Metab.* **29**, 879–883.

Krey, L. C., Butler, W. R. and Knobil, E. (1975). Surgical disconnection of the medial basal hypothalamus and pituitary function in the rhesus monkey. I. Gonadotropin secretion. *Endocrinology* **96**, 1073–1087.

Krohn, P. L. (1962). Review lectures on senescence. II. Heterochronic transplantation in the study of ageing. *Proc. R. Soc. London, Ser. B* **157**, 128–147.

Krohn, P. L. (1964). The reproductive lifespan. *Congr. Int. Riprod. Anim. Fecond. Artif.* **5**, 23–55.

Krølner, B. and Toft, B. (1983). Vertebral bone loss: An unheeded side effect of therapeutic bed rest. *Clin. Sci.* **64**, 537–540.

Kruse-Larsen, C. and Garde, K. (1971). Postmenopausal bleeding: another side-effect of levodopa. *Lancet* **1**, 707–708.

Kupperman, H. S., Wetchler, B. B. and Blatt, M. H. G. (1959). Contemporary therapy of the menopausal syndrome. *JAMA, J. Am. Med. Assoc.* **171**, 1627–1637.

Laing, L. M. (1980). Declining fertility in a religious isolate: The Hutterite population of Alberta, Canada. 1951–1971. *Hum. Biol.* **52**, 288–310.

Laing, S. C., Gosden, R. G. and Fraser, H. M. (1984). Cytogenetic analysis of mouse oocytes after experimental induction of follicular overripening. *J. Reprod. Fertil.* **70**, 387–393.

Land, R. B., de Reviers, M.-M., Thompson, R. and Mauléon, P. (1974). Quantitative physiological studies of genetic variation in the ovarian activity of the rat. *J. Reprod. Fertil.* **38**, 29 –39.

Lang, W. R. and Aponte, G. E. (1967). Gross and microscopic anatomy of the aged female reproductive organs. *Clin. Obstet. Gynecol.* **10**, 454–465.

Lansing, A. I. (1947). A transmissible, cumulative, and reversible factor in aging. *J. Gerontol.* **2**, 228–239.

Larson, L. L. and Foote, R. H. (1972). Uterine blood flow in young and aged rabbits. *Proc. Soc. Exp. Biol. Med.* **141**, 67–69.

Lauritsen, J. G., Bolund, L., Friedrich, U. and Therkelsen, A. J. (1979). Origin of triploidy in spontaneous abortuses. *Ann. Hum. Genet.* **43**, 1–6.

LeBlanc, A. D., Evans, H. J., Johnson, P. C. and Jhingran, S. (1983). Changes in total body calcium balance with exercise in the rat. *J. Appl. Physiol.* **55**, 201–204.

Legan, S. J. and Karsch, F. J. (1975). A daily signal for the LH surge in the rat. *Endocrinology* **96**, 57–62.

Lehrer, S. (1981). Fertility and menopause in blind women. *Fertil. Steril.* **36**, 396–398.

Leridon, H. (1977). "Human Fertility. The Basic Components," pp. 62–67. Univ. of Chicago Press, Chicago, Illinois.

Levine, J. E. and Ramirez, V. D. (1982). Luteinizing hormone-releasing hormone release during the rat estrous cycle and after ovariectomy, as estimated with push-pull cannulae. *Endocrinology* **111**, 1439–1449.

Lévi-Strauss, C. (1966). "Mythologiques: Du Miel aux Cendres." Plon, Paris.

Lightman, S. L., Jacobs, H. S., Maguire, A. K., McGarrick, G. and Jeffcoate, S. L. (1981). Climacteric flushing: Clinical and endocrine response to infusion of naloxone. *Br. J. Obstet. Gynaecol.* **88**, 919–924.

Lindquist, O. and Bengtsson, C. (1979). The effect of smoking on menopausal age. *Maturitas* **1**, 191–199.

Lindquist, O. and Bengtsson, C. (1980). Serum lipids, arterial blood pressure and body weight in relation to the menopause: Results from a population study of women in Göteborg, Sweden. *Scand. J. Clin. Lab. Invest.* **40**, 629–636.

Lindsay, R. and Hart, D. M. (1978). Failure of response of menopausal vasomotor symptoms to clonidine. *Maturitas* **1**, 21–25.

Lindsay, R., Hart, D. M., Aitken, J. M., MacDonald, E. B., Anderson, J. B. and Clarke, A. C. (1976). Long-term prevention of postmenopausal osteoporosis by oestrogen. *Lancet* **1**, 1038–1041.

Lindsay, R., Hart, D. M., MacLean, A., Clarke, A. C., Kraszewski, A. and Garwood, J. (1978). Bone response to termination of oestrogen treatment. *Lancet* **1**, 1325–1327.

Lindsay, R., Hart, D. M., MacLean, A., Garwood, J., Clark, A. C. and Kraszewski, A. (1979). Bone loss during oestriol therapy in postmenopausal women. *Maturitas* **1**, 279–285.

Linnoila, M. and Cooper, R. L. (1976). Reinstatement of vaginal cycles in aged female rats. *J. Pharmacol. Exp. Ther.* **199**, 477–482.

Lintern-Moore, S. and Moore, G. P. M. (1979). The initiation of follicle and oocyte growth in the mouse ovary. *Biol. Reprod.* **20**, 773–778.

Lipschutz, A. (1927). On some fundamental laws of ovarian dynamics. *Biol. Rev. Cambridge Philos. Soc.* **2**, 263–280.

Lloyd, T. and Weisz, J. (1978). Direct inhibition of tyrosine hydroxylase activity by catechol estrogens. *J. Biol. Chem.* **253**, 4841–4843.

Lloyd, T., Weisz, J. and Breakefield, X. O. (1978). The catechol estrogen, 2-hydroxyestradiol, inhibits catechol-O-methyltransferase activity in neuroblastoma cells. *J. Neurochem.* **31**, 245–250.

Lobo, R. A., McCormick, W., Singer, F. and Roy, S. (1984). Depo-medroxyprogesterone acetate compared with conjugated estrogens for the treatment of postmenopausal women. Obstet. Gynec. **63**, 1–5.

Longcope, C. (1971). Metabolic clearance and blood production rates of estrogens in postmenopausal women. *Am. J. Obstet. Gynecol.* **111**, 778–781.

Longcope, C., Layne, D. S. and Tait, J. F. (1968). Metabolic clearance rates and interconversions of estrone and 17β-estradiol in normal males and females. *J. Clin. Invest.* **47**, 93–106.

Longcope, C., Kato, T. and Horton, R. (1969). Conversion of blood androgens to estrogens in normal adult men and women. *J. Clin. Invest.* **48**, 2191–2201.

Longcope, C., Pratt, J. H., Schneider, S. H. and Fineberg, S. E. (1978). Aromatization of androgens by muscle and adipose tissue *in vivo*. *J. Clin. Endocrinol. Metab.* **46**, 146–152.

Longcope, C., Hunter, R. and Franz, C. (1980). Steroid secretion by the postmenopausal ovary. *Am. J. Obstet. Gynecol.* **138**, 564–568.

Lostroh, A. J. and Johnson, R. E. (1966). Amounts of interstitial cell-stimulating hormone and follicle-stimulating hormone required for follicular development, uterine growth and ovulation in the hypophysectomized rat. *Endocrinology* **79**, 991–996.

Louvet, J.-P., Harman, S. M., Schreiber, J. R. and Ross, G. T. (1975). Evidence for a role of androgens in follicular maturation. *Endocrinology* **97**, 366–372.

Lu, J. K. H., Gilman, D. P., Meldrum, D. R., Judd, H. L. and Sawyer, C. H. (1981). Relationship between circulating estrogens and the central mechanisms by which ovarian steroids stimulate luteinizing hormone secretion in aged and young female rats. *Endocrinology* **108**, 836–841.

Lu, K. H., Hopper, B. R., Vargo, T. M. and Yen, S. S. C. (1979). Chronological changes in sex steroid, gonadotropin and prolactin secretion in aging female rats displaying different reproductive states. *Biol. Reprod.* **21**, 193–203.

Luthardt, F. W., Palmer, C. G. and Yu, P.-L. (1973). Chiasma and univalent frequencies in aging female mice. *Cytogenet. Cell Genet.* **12**, 68–79.

Lutjen, P., Trounson, A., Leeton, J., Findlay, J., Wood, C. and Renou, P. (1984). The establishment and maintenance of pregnancy using *in vitro* fertilization and embryo donation in a patient with primary ovarian failure. *Nature (London)* **307**, 174–175.

Lyon, M. F. and Hawker, S. G. (1973). Reproductive lifespan in irradiated and unirradiated chromosomally XO mice. *Genet. Res.* **21**, 185–194.

McCormack, J. T., Plant, T. M., Hess, D. L. and Knobil, E. (1977). The effect of luteinizing hormone releasing hormone (LHRH) antiserum adminstration on gonadotropin secretion in the rhesus monkey. *Endocrinology* **100**, 663–667.

MacCorquodale, D. W., Thayer, S. A. and Doisy, E. A. (1936). The isolation of the principal estrogenic substance of liquor folliculi. *J. Biol. Chem.* **115**, 435–448.

McCoshen, J. A. (1982). In vivo sex differentiation of congeneic germinal cell aplastic gonads. *Am. J. Obstet. Gynecol.* **142**, 83–88.

MacDonald, P. C., Rombaut, R. P. and Siiteri, P. K. (1967). Plasma precursors of estrogen. I. Extent of conversion of plasma Δ^4-androstenedione to estrone in normal males and nonpregnant normal, castrate and adrenalectomized females. *J. Clin. Endocrinol. Metab.* **27**, 1103–1111.

MacDowell, E. C. and Lord, E. M. (1925). The number of corpora lutea in successive mouse pregnancies. *Anat. Rec.* **31**, 131–141.

McGaughey, R. W. (1977). The culture of pig oocytes in minimal medium, and the influence of progesterone and estradiol-17β on meiotic maturation. *Endocrinology* **100**, 39–45.

McKinlay, S., Jefferys, M. and Thompson, B. (1972). An investigation of the age at menopause. *J. Biosocial Sci.* **4**, 161–173.

MacMahon, B. and Worcester, J. (1966). Age at menopause: United States 1960–62. *U.S. Vital Health Stat.*, Ser. II, No. 19.

McNatty, K. P. (1982). Ovarian follicular development from the onset of luteal regression in humans and sheep. *In* "Follicular Maturation and Ovulation" (R. Rolland, E. V. van Hall, S. G. Hillier, K. P. McNatty and J. Schoemaker, eds.), pp. 1–18. Excerpta Medica, Amsterdam.

McNatty, K. P. and Baird, D. T. (1978). Relationship between follicle-stimulating hormone, androstenedione and oestradiol in human follicular fluid. *J. Endocrinol.* **76**, 527–531.

McNatty, K. P., Makris, A., De Grazia, C., Osathanondh, R. and Ryan, K. J. (1979a). The production of progesterone, androgens and estrogens by granulosa cells, theca tissue, and stromal tissue from human ovaries *in vitro*. *J. Clin. Endocrinol. Metab.* **49**, 687–699.

McNatty, K. P., Moore Smith, D., Makris, A., Osathanondh, R. and Ryan, K. J. (1979b). The microenvironment of the human antral follicle: Interrelationships among steroid levels in antral fluid, the population of granulosa cells, and the status of the oocyte *in vivo* and *in vitro*. *J. Clin. Endocrinol. Metab.* **49**, 851–860.

MacRae, K. D. (1981). Health risks of oestrogen therapy. *J. Endocrinol.* **89**, 145P–148P.

Magursky, V., Mesko, M. and Sokolik, L. (1975). Age at the menopause and onset of the climacteric in women of Martin District, Czechoslovakia. *Int. J. Fertil.* **20**, 17–23.

Maibenco, H. C. and Krehbiel, R. H. (1973). Reproductive decline in aged female rats. *J. Reprod. Fertil.* **32**, 121–123.

Makris, A. and Ryan, K. J. (1975). Progesterone, androstenedione, testosterone, estrone, and estradiol synthesis in hamster ovarian follicle cells. *Endocrinology* **96**, 694–701.

Mandl, A. M. and Zuckerman, S. (1951). The numbers of normal and atretic oocytes in unilaterally spayed rats. *J. Endocrinol.* **7**, 112–119.

Maoz, B., Antonovsky, A., Apter, A., Wijsenbeek, H. and Datan, N. (1977). The perception of menopause in five ethnic groups in Israel. *Acta Obstet. Gynecol. Scand., Suppl.* **65**, 69–76.

Marcus, R., Madvig, P. and Young, G. (1984). Age-related changes in parathyroid hormone and parathyroid hormone action in normal humans. *J. Clin. Endocrinol. Metab.* **58**, 223–230.

Marks, R. and Shahrad, P. (1976). Ageing and the effects of estrogens on the skin. *In* "The Menopause: A Guide to Current Research and Practice" (R. J. Beard, ed.), pp. 143–161. MTP Press, Lancaster.

Marshall, D. H., Crilly, R. G. and Nordin, B. E. C. (1977). Plasma androstenedione and oestrone levels in normal and osteoporotic postmenopausal women. *Br. Med. J.* **2**, 1177–1179.

Marshall, D. H., Crilly, R. and Nordin, B. E. C. (1978). The relation between plasma androstenedione and oestrone levels in untreated and corticosteroid-treated post-menopausal women. *Clin. Endocrinol. (Oxford)* **9**, 407–412.

Marshall, F. H. A. (1910). "The Physiology of Reproduction." Longmans, London.

Marshall, F. H. A. and Jolly, W. A. (1906). Contributions to the physiology of mammalian reproduction. Part I. The oestrous cycle in the dog. Part II. The ovary as an organ of internal secretion. *Philos. Trans. R. Soc. London, Ser. B* **198**, 99–141.

Martin, R. H., Balkan, W., Burns, K., Rademaker, A. W., Lin, C. C. and Rudd, N. L. (1983). The chromosome constitution of 1000 human spermatozoa. *Hum. Genet.* **63**, 305–309.

Masters, W. H. and Johnson, V. E. (1966). "Human Sexual Response." Churchill, London.

Mathur, S., Jerath, R. S., Mathur, R. S., Williamson, H. O. and Fudenberg, H. H. (1980a). Serum immunoglobulin levels, autoimmunity and cell-mediated immunity in primary ovarian failure. *J. Reprod. Immunol.* **2**, 83–92.

Mathur, S., Melchers, J. T., III, Ades, E. W., Williamson, H. O. and Fudenberg, H. H. (1980b). Anti-ovarian and anti-lymphocyte antibodies in patients with chronic vaginal Candidiasis. *J. Reprod. Immunol.* **2**, 247–262.

Matsuo, H., Baba, Y., Nair, R. M. G., Arimura, A. and Schally, A. V. (1971). Structure of the porcine LH- and FSH-releasing hormone. I. The proposed amino acid sequence. *Biochem. Biophys. Res. Commun.* **43**, 1334–1339.

Mattingly, R. F. and Huang, W. Y. (1969). Steroidogenesis of the menopausal and postmenopausal ovary. *Am. J. Obstet. Gynecol.* **103**, 679–690.

Mattison, D. R. and Thorgeirsson, S. S. (1978). Smoking and industrial pollution, and their effects on menopause and ovarian cancer. *Lancet* **1**, 187–188.

Mattison, D. R., Evans, M. I., Schwimmer, W. B., White, B. J., Jensen, B. and Schulman, J. D. (1984). Familial prematue ovarian failure. *Am. J. Med. Genet.* (in press.)

Maurer, R. R. and Foote, R. H. (1972). Uterine collagenase and collagen in young and ageing rabbits. *J. Reprod. Fertil.* **30**, 301–304.

Mayer, P. J. (1982). Evolutionary advantage of the menopause. *Hum. Ecol.* **10**, 477–494.

Meade, T. W. (1981). Epidemiology of atheroma and thrombosis. *In* "Haemostasis and Thrombosis'' (A. L. Bloom and D. P. Thomas, eds.), pp. 575–592. Churchill-Livingstone, Edinburgh and London.

Meade, T. W., Haines, A. P., Imeson, J. D., Stirling, Y. and Thompson, S. G. (1983). Menopausal status and haemostatic variables. *Lancet* **1**, 22–24.

Medical Women's Federation (1933). An investigation of the menopause in one thousand women. *Lancet* **1**, 106–108.

Medvedev, Z. A. (1981). On the immortality of the germ line: Genetic and biochemical mechanisms. *Mech. Ageing Dev.* **17**, 331–359.

Meema, H. E. (1966). Menopausal and aging changes in muscle mass and bone mineral content. *J. Bone Joint Surg., Am. Vol.* **48.A**, 1138–1144.

Meites, J., Huang, H. H., Simpkins, J. W. and Steger, R. W. (1982). Central nervous system neurotransmitters during the decline of reproductive activity. *In* ''The Menopause: Clinical, Endocrinological and Pathophysiological Aspects'' (P. Fioretti, L. Martini, G. B. Melis and S. S. C. Yen, eds.), pp. 3–13. Academic Press, New York.

Meldrum, D. R., Tataryn, I. V., Frumar, A. M., Erlik, Y., Lu, K. H. and Judd, H. L. (1980). Gonadotropins, estrogens, and adrenal steroids during the menopausal hot flash. *J. Clin. Endocrinol. Metab.* **50**, 685–689.

Meldrum, D. R., Davidson, B. J., Tataryn, I. V. and Judd, H. L. (1981a). Changes in circulating steroids with aging in postmenopausal women. *Obstet. Gynecol.* (*N.Y.*) **57**, 624–628.

Meldrum, D. R., Erlik, Y., Lu, J. K. H. and Judd, H. L. (1981b). Objectively recorded hot flushes in patients with pituitary insufficiency. *J. Clin. Endocrinol. Metab.* **52**, 684–687.

Merriam, G. R., Brandon, D. D., Kono, S., Davis, S. E., Loriaux, D. L. and Lipsett, M. B. (1980). Rapid metabolic clearance of the catechol estrogen 2-hydroxyestrone. *J. Clin. Endocrinol. Metab.* **51**, 1211–1213.

Metcalf, M. G. (1979). Incidence of ovulatory cycles in women approaching the menopause. *J. Biosocial Sci.* **11**, 39–48.

Metcalf, M. G. (1983). Incidence of ovulation from the menarche to the menopause: observations of 622 New Zealand women. *N.Z. Med. J.* **96**, 645–648.

Metcalf, M. G. and Donald, R. A. (1979). Fluctuating ovarian function in a perimenopausal woman. *N.Z. Med. J.* **89**, 45–47.

Metcalf, M. G. and MacKenzie, J. A. (1980). Incidence of ovulation in young women. *J. Biosocial Sci.* **12**, 345–352.

Metcalf, M. G., Donald, R. A. and Livesey, J. H. (1981a). Classification of menstrual cycles in pre- and postmenopausal women. *J. Endocrinol.* **91**, 1–10.

Metcalf, M. G., Donald, R. A. and Livesey, J. H. (1981b). Pituitary-ovarian function in normal women during the menopausal transition. *Clin. Endocrinol.* (*Oxford*) **14**, 245–255.

Metcalf, M. G., Donald, R. A. and Livesey, J. H. (1982). Pituitary-ovarian function before, during and after the menopause: A longitudinal study. *Clin. Endocrinol.* (*Oxford*) **17**, 489–494.

Michael, R. P. and Bonsall, R. W. (1977). Peri-ovulatory synchronization of behaviour in male and female rhesus monkeys. *Nature* (*London*) **265**, 463–465.

Michael, S. D., Taguchi, O. and Nishizuka, Y. (1981). Changes in hypophyseal hormones associated with accelerated aging and tumorigenesis of the ovaries in neonatally thymectomized mice. *Endocrinology* **108**, 2375–2380.

Mikamo, K. (1968). Mechanism of non-disjunction of meiotic chromosomes and of degeneration of maturation spindles in eggs affected by intrafollicular overripeness. *Experientia* **24**, 75–78.

Mikamo, K. and Hamaguchi, H. (1975). Chromosomal disorder caused by preovulatory overripeness of oocytes. *In* ''Aging Gametes'' (R. J. Blandau, ed.), pp. 72–97. Karger, Basel.

Mikkelsen, M., Poulsen, H., Grinsted, J. and Lange, A. (1980). Non-disjunction in trisomy-21: Study of chromosomal heteromorphisms in 110 families. *Ann. Hum. Genet.* **44**, 17–28.

Milhaud, G., Benezech-Lefevre, M. and Moukhtar, M. S. (1978). Deficiency of calcitonin in age-related osteoporosis. *Biomedicine* **29**, 272–276.

Miller, A. E. and Riegle, G. D. (1980). Serum progesterone during pregnancy and pseudopregnancy and gestation length in the aging rat. *Biol. Reprod.* **22**, 751–758.

Miller, G. J. and Miller, N. E. (1975). Plasma high density lipoprotein concentration and development of ischaemic heart disease. *Lancet* **1**, 16–19.

Miller, J. F., Williamson, E., Glue, J., Gordon, Y. B., Grudzinskas, J. G. and Sykes, A. (1980). Fetal loss after implantation. *Lancet* **2**, 554–556.

Miller, M. E. and Chatten, J. (1967). Ovarian changes in ataxia telangiectasia. *Acta Paediatr. Scand.* **56**, 559–561.

Mintz, B. and Russell, E. S. (1957). Gene-induced embryological modifications of primordial germ cells in the mouse. *J. Exp. Zool.* **134**, 207–237.

Mittwoch, U. and Delhanty, J. D. A. (1972). Inhibition of mitosis in human triploid cells. *Nature (London), New Biol.* **238**, 11–13.

Mizoguchi, H. and Dukelow, W. R. (1981). Fertilizability of ova from young or old hamsters after spontaneous or induced ovulation. *Fertil. Steril.* **35**, 79–83.

Mobbs, C. V., Flurkey, K., Gee, D. M., Yamamoto, K., Sinha, Y. N. and Finch, C. E. (1984). Estradiol-induced adult anovulatory syndrome in female C57BL/6J mice: Age-like neuroendocrine, but not ovarian, impairments. *Biol. Reprod.* **30**, 550–553.

Molnar, G. W. (1975). Body temperatures during menopausal hot flushes. *J. Appl. Physiol.* **38**, 499–503.

Monk, M. and McLaren, A. (1981). X-chromosome activity in foetal germ cells of the mouse. *J. Embryol. Exp. Morphol.* **63**, 75–84.

Moon, Y. S., Tsang, B. K., Simpson, C. and Armstrong, D. T. (1978). 17β-estradiol biosynthesis in cultured granulosa and theca cells of human ovarian follicles: Stimulation by follicle-stimulating hormone. *J. Clin. Endocrinol. Metab.* **47**, 263–267.

Moor, R. M. (1974). The ovarian follicle of the sheep: Inhibition of oestrogen secretion by luteinizing hormone. *J. Endocrinol.* **61**, 455–463.

Moor, R. M. (1977). Sites of steroid production in ovine Graafian follicles in culture. *J. Endocrinol.* **73**, 143–150.

Moore, C. R. and Price, D. (1932). Gonad hormone functions, and the reciprocal influence between gonads and hypophysis with its bearing on the problem of sex hormone antagonism. *Am. J. Anat.* **50**, 13–71.

Mori, T., Fujita, Y., Nihnobu, K., Ezaki, Y., Kubo, K. and Nishimura, T. (1982). Steroidogenesis *in vitro* by human ovarian follicles during the process of atresia. *Clin. Endocrinol. (Oxford)* **16**, 391–400.

Morimoto, S., Tsuji, M., Okada, Y., Onishi, T. and Kumahara, Y. (1980). The effect of oestrogens on human calcitonin secretion after calcium infusions in elderly female subjects. *Clin. Endocrinol. (Oxford)* **13**, 135–143.

Morrell, M. J., Dixen, J. M., Carter, C. S. and Davidson, J. M. (1984). The influence of age and cycling status on sexual arousability in women. *Am. J. Obstet. Gynecol.* **148**, 66–71.

Morrison, J. C., Givens, J. R., Wiser, W. L. and Fish, S. A. (1975). Mumps oophoritis: A cause of premature menopause. *Fert. Steril.* **26**, 655–659.

Mosko, S. S., Erickson, G. F. and Moore, R. Y. (1980). Dampened circadian rhythms in reproductively senescent female rats. *Behav. Neural Biol.* **28**, 1–14.

Mulley, G., Mitchell, J. R. A. and Tattersall, R. B. (1977). Hot flushes after hypophysectomy. *Br. Med. J.* **2**, 1062.

Murphy, E. D. (1972). Hyperplastic and early neoplastic changes in the ovaries of mice after genic deletion of germ cells. *J. Natl. Cancer Inst. (U.S.)* **48**, 1283–1295.

172

References

Naeye, R. L. (1979). The duration of maternal cigarette smoking, fetal and placental disorders. *Early Hum. Dev.* **3**, 229–237.

Naeye, R. L. (1983). Maternal age, obstetric complications, and the outcome of pregnancy. *Obstet. Gynecol. (N.Y.)* **61**, 210–216.

Naftolin, F., Ryan, K. J., Davies, I. J., Reddy, V. V., Flores, F., Petro, Z., Kuhn, M., White, R. J., Takaoka, Y. and Wolin, L. (1975). The formation of estrogens by central neuroendocrine tissues. *Recent Prog. Horm. Res.* **31**, 295–315.

Nass, T. E., Lapolt, P. S. and Lu, J. K. H. (1982). Effects of prolonged caging with fertile males on reproductive functions in aging female rats. *Biol. Reprod.* **27**, 609–615.

Nathan, E., Knoth, M., and Nilsson, B. O. (1978). Scanning electron microscopy of the effect of short-term hormonal therapy on postmenopausal endometrium. *Upsala J. Med. Sci.* **83**, 175–183.

Naylor, A. F. and Warburton, D. (1979). Sequential analysis of spontaneous abortion. II. Collaborative study data show that gravidity determines a very substantial rise in risk. *Fertil. Steril.* **31**, 282–286.

Nelson, J. F., Latham, K. R. and Finch, C. E. (1975). Plasma testosterone levels in C57BL/6J male mice: Effects of age and disease. *Acta Endocrinol. (Copenhagen)* **80**, 744–752.

Nelson, J. F. Felicio, L. S., Randall, P. K., Sims, C. and Finch, C. E. (1982). A longitudinal study of estrous cyclicity in aging C57BL/6J mice. I. Cycle frequency, length and vaginal cytology. *Biol. Reprod.* **27**, 327–339.

Nelson, J. F., Gosden, R. G. and Felicio, L. S. (1985). Effect of dietary restriction on estrous cyclicity, follicular reserves and the post-castration rise of LH in aging C57BL/6J mice. *Biol. Reprod.* (in press).

Nikkilä, E. A. (1978). Metabolic and endocrine control of plasma high density lipoprotein concentration. *In* "High Density Lipoproteins and Atherosclerosis" (A. M. Gotto, Jr., N. E. Miller and M. F. Oliver, eds.), pp. 177–192. Elsevier/North-Holland, Amsterdam.

Nilsson, L., Wikland, M. and Hamberger, L. (1982). Recruitment of an ovulatory follicle in the human following follicle-ectomy and luteectomy. *Fertil. Steril.* **37**, 30–34.

Nichols, K. C., Schenkel, L. and Benson, H. (1984). 17β-estradiol for postmenopausal estrogen replacement therapy. *Obstet. Gynecol. Survey* **39**, 230–245.

Nimrod, A. and Ryan, K. J. (1975). Aromatization of androgens by human abdominal and breast fat tissue. *J. Clin. Endocrinol. Metab.* **40**, 367–372.

Nishimura, H. and Shikata, A. (1960). High embryonic mortality of the mouse fetuses from the elderly primigravid mothers. *Okajimas Folia Anat. Jpn.* **36**, 151–154.

Nishizuka, Y., Taguchi, O., Sakaguchi, S., Takahashi, T., Kojima, A. and Sakakura, T. (1981). Ovarian and testicular dysgenesis in immunodeficient mice: Its genesis and autoimmune nature. *In* "Development and Function of Reproductive Organs" (A. G. Byskov and H. Peters, eds.), I.C.S. No. 559, pp. 250–257. Excerpta Medica, Amsterdam.

Nordin, B. E. C., MacGregor, J. and Smith, D. A. (1966). The incidence of osteoporosis in normal women: Its relation to age and the menopause. *Q. J. Med.* [N.S.] **35**, 25–38.

Nordin, B. E. C., Horsman, A., Crilly, R. G., Marshall, D. H. and Simpson, M. (1980b). Treatment of spinal osteoporosis in postmenopausal women. *Br. Med. J.* (280), 451–454.

Nordin, B. E. C., Horsman, A., Crilly, R. G., Marshall, D. H. and Simpson, M. (1980b). Treatment of spinal osteoporosis in postmenopausal women. *Br. Med. J.*, (280), 451–454.

Norman, R. L., Resko, J. A. and Spies, H. G. (1976). The anterior hypothalamus: How it affects gonadotropin secretion in the rhesus monkey. *Endocrinology* **99**, 59–71.

Notelovitz, M. (1982). Carbohydrate metabolism in relation to hormonal replacement therapy. *Acta Obstet. Gynecol. Scand., Suppl.* **106**, 51–56.

Notelovitz, M., Kitchens, C. S. and Ware, M. D. (1984). Coagulation and fibrinolysis in estrogen-treated surgically menopausal women. *Obstet. Gynec.* **63**, 621–625.

Nussbaum, M. (1880). Zur Differenzierung des Geschlechts im Theirreich. *Arch. Mikrosk. Anat.* **18**, 1–120.

O'Dea, J. P. K., Wieland, R. G., Hallberg, M. C., Llerena, L. A., Zorn, E. M. and Genuth, S. M. (1979). Effect of dietary weight loss on sex steroid binding, sex steroids, and gonadotropins in obese postmenopausal women. *J. Lab. Clin. Med.* **93**, 1004–1008.

Odell, W. D. and Swerdloff, R. S. (1968). Progestogen-induced luteinizing and follicle stimulating hormone surge in postmenopausal women: A simulated ovulatory peak. *Proc. Natl. Acad. Sci. U.S.A.* **61**, 529–536.

Oliver, M. F. and Boyd, G. S. (1959). Effect of bilateral ovariectomy on coronary-artery disease and serum lipid levels. *Lancet* **2**, 690–694.

Oźdzeński, W. (1967). Observations on the origin of primordial germ cells in the mouse. *Zool. Pol.* **17**, 367–379.

Page, R. D. and Butcher, R. L. (1982). Follicular and plasma patterns of steroids in young and old rats during normal and prolonged estrous cycles. *Biol. Reprod.* **27**, 383–392.

Page, R. D., Kirkpatrick-Keller, D. and Butcher, R. L. (1983). Role of age and length of oestrous cycle in alteration of the oocyte and intrauterine environment in the rat. *J. Reprod. Fertil.* **69**, 23–28.

Parfitt, A. M. (1983). Dietary risk factors for age-related bone loss and fractures. *Lancet* **2**, 1181–1185.

Parkening, T. A. and Soderwall, A. L. (1973). Delayed embryonic development and implantation in senescent golden hamsters. *Biol. Reprod.* **8**, 427–434.

Parkening, T. A., Collins, T. J. and Smith, E. R. (1980). Plasma and pituitary concentrations of LH, FSH and prolactin in aged female C57BL/6 mice. *J. Reprod. Fertil.* **58**, 377–386.

Parker, C. R., Jr. and Porter, J. C. (1984). Luteinizing hormone-releasing hormone and thyrotropin-releasing hormone in the hypothalamus of women: Effects of age and reproductive status. *J. Clin. Endocrinol. Metab.* **58**, 488–491.

Parkes, A. S. (1937). Source of androgenic and oestrogenic substances of the urine. *Lancet* **2**, 902–903.

Parsons, P. A. (1964). Parental age and the offspring. *Q. Rev. Biol.* **39**, 258–275.

Paterson, M. E. L. (1982). A randomized double-blind cross-over trial into the effect of nor-ethisterone on climacteric symptoms and biochemical profiles. *Br. J. Obstet. Gynecol.* **89**, 464–472.

Patwardhan, V. V. and Lanthier, A. (1977). Pathways for the biosynthesis of oestradiol in the rabbit ovarian follicle *in vitro*. *J. Endocrinol.* **75**, 445–446.

Pedersen, T. (1970). Determination of follicle growth rate in the ovary of the immature mouse. *J. Reprod. Fertil.* **21**, 81–93.

Pedersen, T. and Peters, H. (1968). Proposal for a classification of oocytes and follicles in the mouse ovary. *J. Reprod. Fertil.* **17**, 555–557.

Peluso, J. J., Steger, R. W., Huang, H. and Meites, J. (1979). Pattern of follicular growth and steroidogenesis in the ovary of aging cycling rats. *Exp. Aging Res.* **5**, 319–333.

Peng, M. and Huang, H. (1972). Aging of the hypothalamic-pituitary-ovarian function in the rat. *Fertil. Steril.* **23**, 535–542.

Peng, M. T., Chuong, C. F. and Peng, Y. M. (1977). Lordosis response of senile female rats. *Neuroendocrinology* **24**, 317–324.

Penrose, L. S. (1933). The relative effects of paternal and maternal age in mongolism. *J. Genet.* **27**, 219–224.

Penrose, L. S. (1961). Mongolism. *Br. Med. Bull.* **17**, 184–189.

Perry, J. S. (1953). The reproduction of the African elephant *Loxodonta africana*. *Philos. Trans. R. Soc. London, Ser. B* **237** 93–149.

Peters, H. (1969). The effect of radiation in early life on the morphology and reproductive function of the mouse ovary. *Adv. Reprod. Physiol.* **4**, 149–185.

Peters, H. (1970). Migration of gonocytes into the mammalian gonad and their differentiation. *Philos. Trans. R. Soc. London, Ser. B* **259**, 91–101.

Peters, H., Byskov, A. G., Himelstein-Braw, R. and Faber, M. (1975). Follicular growth: The basic event in the mouse and human ovary. *J. Reprod. Fertil.* **45**, 559–566.

Pfeffer, R. I., Whipple, G. H., Kurosaki, T. T. and Chapman, J. M. (1978). Coronary risk and estrogen use in postmenopausal women. *Am. J. Epidemiol.* **107**, 479–497.

Pike, M. C., Henderson, B. E., Krailo, M. D., Duke, A. and Roy, S. (1983). Breast cancer in young women and use of oral contraceptives: Possible modifying effect of formulation and age at use. *Lancet* **2**, 926–930.

Pittenger, D. (1973). An exponential model of female sterility. *Demography* **10**, 113–121.

Pohl, C. R., Richardson, D. W., Hutchison, J. S., Germak, J. A. and Knobil, E. (1983). Hypophysiotropic signal frequency and the functioning of the pituitary-ovarian system in the rhesus monkey. *Endocrinology* **112**, 2076–2080.

Polani, P. E. (1974). Chromosomal and other genetic influences on birth weight variation. *Ciba Found. Symp.* [N.S.] **27**, 127–160.

Polani, P. E. and Jagiello, G. M. (1976). Chiasmata, meiotic univalents, and age in relation to aneuploid imbalance in mice. *Cytogenet. Cell Genet.* **16**, 505–529.

Polednak, A. P. (1976). Paternal age in relation to selected birth defects. *Hum. Biol.* **48**, 727–739.

Post, J. B. (1971). Ages at menarche and menopause: Some mediaeval authorities. *Popul. Stud.* **25**, 83–87.

Pott, P. (1775). An ovarian hernia. *In* "The Chirurgical Works," pp. 791–792. London.

Psychoyos, A. (1973). Endocrine control of egg implantation. *In* "Handbook of Physiology" (R. O. Greep and E. B. Astwood, eds.), Sect. 7, Vol. II, Part 2, pp. 187–215. Am. Physiol. Soc., Washington, D.C.

Pumpianski, R. (1967). Age at natural menopause. *Harefuah* **77**, 513–516.

Punnonen, R. (1972). Effect of castration and peroral estrogen therapy on the skin. *Acta Obstet. Gynecol. Scand., Suppl.* **21**, 1–44.

Punnonen, R., Vilska, S., Grönroos, M. and Rauramo, L. (1980). The vaginal absorption of oestrogens in post-menopausal women. *Maturitas* **2**, 321–326.

Quadri, S. K., Kledzik, G. S. and Meites, J. (1973). Reinitiation of estrous cycles in old constant-estrous rats by central-acting drugs. *Neuroendocrinology* **11**, 248–255.

Rao, M. C., Midgley, A. R., Jr. and Richards, J. S. (1978). Hormonal regulation of ovarian cellular proliferation. *Cell* **14**, 71–78.

Rattray, P. V. (1977). Nutrition and reproductive efficiency. *In* "Reproduction in Domestic Animals" (H. H. Cole and P. T. Cupps, eds.), 3rd ed., pp. 553–575. Academic Press, New York.

Read, S. G. (1982). The distribution of Down's syndrome. *J. Ment. Defic. Res.* **26**, 215–227.

Reader, S. C. J., Robertson, W. R. and Diczfalusy, E. (1983). Microheterogeneity of luteinizing hormone in pituitary glands from women of pre- and postmenopausal age. *Clin. Endocrinol. (Oxford)* **19**, 355–363.

Rebar, R. W., Erickson, G. F. and Yen, S. S. C. (1982). Idiopathic premature ovarian failure: Clinical and endocrine characteristics. *Fertil. Steril.* **37**, 35–41.

Recker, R. R., Saville, P. D. and Heaney, R. P. (1977). Effect of estrogens and calcium carbonate on bone loss in postmenopausal women. *Ann. Intern. Med.* **87**, 649–655.

Record, R. G. (1961). Anencephalus in Scotland. *Br. J. Prev. Soc. Med.* **15**, 93–105.

Resseguie, L. J. (1974). Pregnancy wastage and age of mother among the Amish. *Hum. Biol.* **46**, 633–639.

Reyes, F. I., Koh, K. S. and Faiman, C. (1976). Fertility in women with gonadal dysgenesis. *Am. J. Obstet. Gynecol.* **126**, 668–670.

Reyes, F. I., Winter, J. S. D. and Faiman, C. (1977). Pituitary-ovarian relationships preceding the menopause. I. A cross-sectional study of serum follicle stimulating hormone, luteinizing hormone, prolactin, estradiol and progesterone levels. *Am. J. Obstet. Gynecol.* **129,** 557 –564.

Richards, J. S. (1979). Hormonal control of ovarian follicular development. A 1978 perspective. *Recent Prog. Horm. Res.* **35,** 343–368.

Riemersma, R. A. (1984). Coronary artery disease: Raised cholesterol or triglycerides? *Int. J. Cardiol.* **5,** 193–194.

Riggs, B. L. and Melton, L. J., III (1983). Evidence for two distinct syndromes of involutional osteoporosis. *Am. J. Med.* **75,** 899–901.

Riggs, B. L., Jowsey, J., Kelly, P. J., Jones, J. D. and Maher, F. T. (1969). Effect of sex hormones on bone in primary osteoporosis. *J. Clin. Invest.* **48,** 1065–1072.

Riggs, B. L., Seeman, E., Hodgson, S. F., Taves, D. R. and O'Fallon, W. M. (1982). Effect of the fluoride/calcium regimen on vertebral fracture occurrence in postmenopausal osteoporosis. *N. Engl. J. Med.* **306,** 446–450.

Roberts, C. J. and Lowe, C. R. (1975). Where have all the conceptions gone? *Lancet* **1,** 498–499.

Roberts, D. F. (1979). Genetics and ageing in man. *J. Biosocial Sci., Suppl.* **6,** 177–195.

Roberts, K. D., Rochefort, J. G., Blean, G. and Chapdelaine, A. (1980). Plasma estrone sulfate levels in postmenopausal women. *Steroids* **35,** 179–187.

Roberts, R. C. (1961). The lifetime growth and reproduction of selected strains of mice. *Heredity* **16,** 369–381.

Rodman, T. C. (1971). Chromatid disjunction in unfertilized aging oocytes. *Nature (London)* **233,** 191–192.

Roecker, G. O. and Huether, C. A. (1983). An analysis for paternal age effect in Ohio's Down syndrome births, 1970–1980. *Am. J. Hum. Genet.* **35,** 1297–1306.

Roger, M., Nahoul, K., Scholler, R. and Bagrel, D. (1980). Evolution with ageing of four plasma androgens in postmenopausal women. *Maturitas* **2,** 171–177.

Rose, D. P. and Davis, T. E. (1977). Ovarian function in patients receiving adjuvant chemotherapy for breast cancer. *Lancet* **1,** 1174–1176.

Rosenberg, L., Hennekens, C. H., Rosner, B., Belanger, C., Rothman, K. J. and Speizer, F. E. (1981). Early menopause and the risk of myocardial infarction. *Am. J. Obstet. Gynecol.* **139,** 47–51.

Ross, C. A. C. (1978). Post-menopausal vaginitis. *J. Med. Microbiol.* **11,** 209–210.

Ross, R. K., Paganini-Hill, A., Mack, T. M., Arthur, M. and Henderson, B. E. (1981). Menopausal oestrogen therapy and protection from death from ischaemic heart disease. *Lancet* **1,** 858–860.

Royal College of General Practitioners' Oral Contraception Study (1977). Mortality among oral contraceptive users. *Lancet* **2,** 727–731.

Royal College of General Practitioners' Oral Contraception Study (1978). Reduction in incidence of rheumatoid arthritis associated with oral contraceptives. *Lancet* **1,** 569–571.

Rumery, R. E. and Eddy, E. M. (1974). Scanning electron microscopy of the fimbriae and ampullae of rabbit oviducts. *Anat. Rec.* **178,** 83–102.

Russell, P. and Altschuler, G. (1975). The ovarian dysgenesis of trisomy 18. *Pathology* **7,** 149–155.

Russell, W. T. (1936). Statistical study of the sex ratio at birth. *J. Hyg.* **36,** 381–401.

Ryan, K. J. (1959). Biological aromatization of steroids. *J. Biol. Chem.* **234,** 268–272.

Ryan, K. J. and Petro, Z. (1966). Steroid biosynthesis by human ovarian granulosa and thecal cells. *J. Clin. Endocrinol. Metab.* **26,** 46–52.

Ryan, K. J., Petro, Z. and Kaiser, J. (1968). Steroid formation by isolated and recombined ovarian granulosa and thecal cells. *J. Clin. Endocrinol. Metab.* **28,** 355–358.

Sanders, D. and Bancroft, J. (1982). Hormones and the sexuality of women—the menstrual cycle. *Clin. Endocrinol. Metab.* **11,** 639–659.

Sarkar, D. K., Chiappa, S. A., Fink, G. and Sherwood, N. M. (1976). Gonadotropin-releasing hormone surge in pro-oestrous rats. *Nature (London)* **264**, 461–463.

Scaramuzzi, R. J. and Radford, H. M. (1983). Factors regulating ovulation rate in the ewe. *J. Reprod. Fertil.* **69**, 353–367.

Schaeffer, J. M. and Hsueh, A. J. W. (1979). 2-hydroxyestradiol interaction with dopamine receptor binding in rat anterior pituitary. *J. Biol. Chem.* **254**, 5606–5608.

Schaub, M. C. (1964–1965). Changes of collagen in the aging and in the pregnant uterus of white rats. *Gerontologia* **10**, 137–145.

Schwartz, D., MacDonald, P. D. M. and Heuchel, V. (1980). Fecundability, coital frequency and the viability of ova. *Popul. Stud.* **34**, 397–400.

Schwartz, E., Wiedemann, E., Simon, S. and Schiffer, M. (1969). Estrogenic antagonism of metabolic effects of administered growth hormone. *J. Clin. Endocrinol. Metab.* **29**, 1176–1181.

Scragg, R. F. R. (1973). Menopause and reproductive span in rural Niugini. *In* "Proceedings of the Annual Symposium of the Papua New Guinea Medical Society, Port Moresby," pp. 126–144.

Selvin, S. and Janerich, D. T. (1971). Four factors influencing birthweight. *Br. J. Prev. Soc. Med.* **25**, 12–16.

Semmens, J. P. and Wagner, G. (1982). Estrogen deprivation and vaginal function in postmenopausal women. *JAMA, J. Am. Med. Assoc.* **248**, 445–448.

Shamonki, I. M., Frumar, A. M., Tataryn, I. V., Meldrum, D. R., Davidson, B. H., Parthemore, J. G., Judd, H. L. and Deftos, L. J. (1980). Age-related changes of calcitonin secretion in female *J. Clin. Endocrinol. Metab.* **50**, 437–439.

Sherman, B. M., West, J. H. and Korenman, S. G. (1976). The menopausal transition: Analysis of LH, FSH, estradiol and progesterone concentrations during menstrual cycles of older women. *J. Clin. Endocrinol. Metab.* **42**, 629–636.

Sherman, B. M., Wallace, R. B. and Treloar, A. E. (1979). The menopausal transition: Endocrinological and epidemiological considerations. *J. Biosocial Sci., Suppl.* **6**, 19–35.

Sherman, B. M., Wallace, R. B., Bean, J. A. and Schlabaugh, L. (1981). Relationship of body weight to menarcheal and menopausal age: Implications for breast cancer risk. *J. Clin. Endocrinol. Metab.* **52**, 488–493.

Shivers, B. D., Harlan, R. E., Morrell, J. I. and Pfaff, D. W. (1983). Absence of oestradiol concentration in cell nuclei of LH-RH-immunoreactive neurones. *Nature (London)* **304**, 345–347.

Short, R. V. (1962). Steroids in the follicular fluid and the corpus luteum of the mare. A "two-cell type" theory of ovarian steroid synthesis. *J. Endocrinol.* **24**, 59–63.

Short, R. V. (1976). The evolution of human reproduction. *Proc. R. Soc. London* **195**, 3–24.

Sigler, A. T., Cohen, B. H., Lilienfeld, A. M., Westlake, J. E. and Hetznecker, W. H. (1967). Reproductive and marital experience of parents of children with Down's syndrome (mongolism). *J. Pediatr.* **70**, 608–614.

Siiteri, P. K. (1981). Extraglandular oestrogen formation and serum binding of oestradiol: relationship to cancer. *J. Endocrinol.* **89**, 119P–129P.

Siiteri, P. K. and MacDonald, P. C. (1973). Role of extraglandular estrogen in human endocrinology. *In* "Handbook of Physiology" (R. O. Greep and E. B. Astwood, eds.), Sect. 7, Vol. II, Part 1, pp. 615–629. Am. Physiol. Soc., Washington, D.C.

Simpkins, J. W., Advis, J. P., Hodson, C. A. and Meites, J. (1979). Blockade of steroid-induced luteinizing hormone release by selective depletion of anterior hypothalamic norepinephrine activity. *Endocrinology* **104**, 506–509.

Simpson, J. L. (1983). Genetic forms of gonadal dysgenesis in 46,XX and 46,XY individuals. *Sem. Reprod. Endocrinol.* **1**, 93–100.

Singh, L. and Ahuja, S. (1980). Trend of menopause among the women of Punjab. *Anthropol. Anz.* **38**, 297–300.

Slaunwhite, W. R., Jr., Kirdani, R. Y. and Sandberg, A. A. (1973). Metabolic aspects of estrogens in man. *In* "Handbook of Physiology" (R. O. Greep and E. B. Astwood, eds.), Sect. 7, Vol. II, Part 1, pp. 485–523. Am. Physiol. Soc., Washington, D.C.

Smith, A. F. (1975). Ultrastructure of the uterine epithelium at the time of implantation in ageing mice. *J. Reprod. Fertil.* **42**, 183–185.

Smith, G. F. and Berg, J. M. (1976). "Down's Anomaly," 2nd ed. Churchill-Livingstone, Edinburgh and London.

Smith, M. A., Wilson, J. and Price, W. H. (1982). Bone demineralization in patients with Turner's syndrome. *J. Med. Genet.* **19**, 100–103.

Smith, P. (1972). Age changes in the female urethra. *Br. J. Urol.* **44**, 667–676.

Smith, Q. T. and Allison, D. J. (1966). Changes of collagen content in skin, femur and uterus of 17β-estradiol benzoate-treated rats. *Endocrinology* **79**, 486–492.

Smuk, M. and Schwers, J. (1977). Aromatization of androstenedione by human adult liver *in vitro*. *J. Clin. Endocrinol. Metab.* **45**, 1009–1012.

Soberon, J., Calderon, J. J. and Goldzieher, J. W. (1966). Relation of parity to age at menopause. *Am. J. Obstet. Gynecol.* **96**, 96–100.

Soderwall, A. L., Kent, H. A., Turbyfill, C. L. and Britenbaker, A. I. (1960). Variation in gestation length and litter size of the golden hamster (*Mesocricetus auratus*). *J. Gerontol.* **15**, 246–248.

Sopelak, V. M. and Butcher, R. L. (1982). Contribution of the ovary versus hypothalamus-pituitary to termination of estrous cycles in aging rats using ovarian transplants. *Biol. Reprod.* **27**, 29–37.

Southren, A. L., Olivo, J., Gordon, G. G., Vittek, J., Brener, J. and Rafii, F. (1974). The conversion of androgens to estrogens in hyperthyroidism. *J. Clin. Endocrinol. Metab.* **38**, 207–214.

Speed, R. M. (1977). The effects of ageing on the meiotic chromosomes of male and female mice. *Chromosoma* **63**, 241–254.

Speed, R. M. and Chandley, A. C. (1983). Meiosis in the foetal mouse ovary. II. Oocyte development and age-related aneuploidy. Does a production line exist? *Chromosoma* **88**, 184–189.

Spilman, C. H., Larson, L. L., Concannon, P. W. and Foote, R. H. (1972). Ovarian function during pregnancy in young and aged rabbits: Temporal relationship between fetal death and corpus luteum regression. *Biol. Reprod.* **7**, 223–230.

Steinach, E. and Kun, H. (1937). Transformation of male sex hormones into a substance with the action of a female hormone. *Lancet* **2**, 845.

Sternberg, W. H. (1949). The morphology, androgenic function, hyperplasia and tumours of the human ovarian hilus cells. *Am. J. Pathol.* **25**, 493–521.

Stevenson, J. C., Abeyasekera, G., Hillyard, C. J., Phang, K. G., MacIntyre, I., Campbell, S., Townsend, P. T., Young, O. and Whitehead, M. I. (1981). Calcitonin and the calcium-regulating hormones in post-menopausal women: Effect of oestrogens. *Lancet* **1**, 693–695.

Strathy, J. H., Coulam, C. B. and Spelsberg, T. C. (1982). Comparison of estrogen receptors in human premenopausal and postmenopausal uteri: Indication of biologically inactive receptor in postmenopausal uteri. *Am. J. Obstet. Gynecol.* **142**, 372–382.

Sturdee, D. W., Wilson, K. A., Pipili, E. and Crocker, A. D. (1978). Physiological aspects of menopausal hot flush. *Br. Med. J.* **2**, 79–80.

Sugawara, S. and Mikamo, K. (1983). Absence of correlation between univalent formation and meiotic non-disjunction in aged female Chinese hamsters. *Cytogenet. Cell Genet.* **35**, 34–40.

Suntzeff, V., Cowdry, E. V. and Hixon, B. B. (1962). Influence of maternal age on offspring in mice. *J. Gerontol.* **17**, 2–7.

Szentágothai, J., Flerkó, B., Mess, B. and Halász, B. (1962). "Hypothalamic Control of the Anterior Pituitary." Akadémiai Kiadó, Budapest.

Tait, J. F. and Horton, R. (1966). The *in vivo* estimation of blood production and interconversion rates of androstenedione and testosterone and the calculation of their secretion rates. *In* "Steroid Dynamics" (G. Pincus, T. Nakao and J. F. Tait, eds.), pp. 393–424. Academic Press, New York.

Talbert, G. B. (1977). The aging of the reproductive system. *In* "Handbook of the Biology of Aging" (C. E. Finch and L. Hayflick, eds.), pp. 318–356. Van Nostrand-Reinhold, Princeton, New Jersey.

Talbert, G. B. and Krohn, P. L. (1966). Effect of maternal age on viability of ova and uterine support of pregnancy in mice. *J. Reprod. Fertil.* **11**, 399–406.

Tam, P. P. L. and Snow, M. H. L. (1981). Proliferation and migration of primordial germ cells during compensatory growth in mouse embryos. *J. Embryol. Exp. Morphol.* **64**, 133–147.

Tanner, J. M. (1978). "Foetus into Man." Open Books, London.

Tataryn, I. V., Meldrum, D. R., Lu, K. H., Frumar, A. M. and Judd, H. L. (1979). LH, FSH and skin temperature during the menopausal hot flash. *J. Clin. Endocrinol. Metab.* **49**, 152–154.

Tataryn, I. V., Lomax, P., Bajorek, J. G., Chesarek, W., Meldrum, D. R. and Judd, H. L. (1980). Postmenopausal hot flushes: A disorder of thermoregulation. *Maturitas* **2**, 101–107.

Tease, C. (1982). Similar dose-related chromosome non-disjunction in young and old female mice after X-irradiation. *Mutat. Res.* **95**, 287–296.

Tejasen, T. and Everett, J. W. (1967). Surgical analysis of the preoptico-tuberal pathway controlling ovulatory release of gonadotropins in the rat. *Endocrinology* **81**, 1387–1396.

Terranova, P. F. (1981). Steroidogenesis in experimentally induced atretic follicles of the hamster: A shift from estradiol to progesterone synthesis. *Endocrinology* **108**, 1885–1890.

Tho, P. T. and McDonough, P. G. (1982). Precocious ovarian failure. *In* "The Menopause: Clinical, Endocrinological and Pathophysiological Aspects" (P. Fioretti, L. Martini, G. B. Melis and S. S. C. Yen, eds.), Serono Symp. No. 39, pp. 351–370. Academic Press, New York.

Thompson, B., Hart, S. A. and Durno, D. (1973). Menopausal age and symptomatology in a general practice. *J. Biosocial Sci.* **5**, 71–82.

Thung, P. J. (1961). Ageing changes in the ovary. *In* "Structural Aspects of Ageing" (G. H. Bourne, ed.), pp. 110–142. Pitman, London.

Tietze, C. (1957). Reproductive span and rate of reproduction among Hutterite women. *Fertil. Steril.* **8**, 89–97.

Tilt, E. J. (1857). "The Change of Life in Health and Disease." Churchill, London.

Tobert, J. A. (1976). A study of the possible role of prostaglandins in decidualization using a novel surgical method for the instillation of fluids into the rat uterine lumen. *J. Reprod. Fertil.* **47**, 391–393.

Treloar, A. E. (1974). Menarche, menopause and intervening fecundability. *Hum. Biol.* **46**, 89–107.

Treloar, A. E. (1981). Menstrual cyclicity and the pre-menopause. *Maturitas* **3**, 249–264.

Treloar, A. E., Boynton, R. E., Behn, B. G. and Brown, B. W. (1967). Variation of the human menstrual cycle through reproductive life. *Int. J. Fertil.* **12**, 77–126.

Trouillas, J., Girod, C., Sassolas, G., Claustrat, B., L héritier, M., Dubois, M. P. and Goutelle, A. (1981). Human pituitary gonadotropic adenoma; histological, immunocytochemical, and ultrastructural and hormonal studies in eight cases. *J. Pathol.* **135**, 315–336.

Twomey, L. and Taylor, J. (1983). Non-hormonal treatment of osteoporosis. *Br. Med. J.* (287), 215.

Twomey, L., Taylor, J. and Furniss, B. (1983). Age changes in the bone density and structure of the lumbar vertebral column. *J. Anat.* **136**, 15–25.

Tyrey, L. (1980). Δ^9-tetrahydrocannabinol: A potent inhibitor of episodic luteinizing hormone secretion. *J. Pharmacol. Exp. Ther.* **213**, 306–308.

Uilenbroek, J. T. J. and Richards, J. S. (1979). Ovarian follicular development during the rat estrous cycle: Gonadotropin receptors and follicular responsiveness. *Biol. Reprod.* **20**, 1159–1165.

Uilenbroek, J. T. J., Woutersen, P. J. A. and van der Schoot, P. (1980). Atresia of preovulatory follicles: Gonadotropin binding and steroidogenic activity. *Biol. Reprod.* **23**, 219–229.

van Keep, P. A. and Humphrey, M. (1976). Psycho-social aspects of the climacteric. *In* "Consensus on Menopause Research" (P. A. van Keep, R. B. Greenblatt and M. Albeaux-Fernet, eds.), pp. 5–8. MTP Press, Lancaster.

van Keep, P. A., Brand, P. C. and Lehert, P. (1979). Factors affecting the age at menopause. *J. Biosocial Sci., Suppl.* **6**, 37–55.

van Look, P. F. A., Lothian, H., Hunter, W. M., Michie, E. A. and Baird, D. T. (1977). Hypothalamic-pituitary-ovarian function in perimenopausal women. *Clin. Endocrinol. (Oxford)* **7**, 13–31.

van Look, P. F. A., Hunter, W. M., Fraser, I. S. and Baird, D. T. (1978). Impaired estrogen-induced luteinizing hormone release in young women with anovulatory dysfunctional uterine bleeding. *J. Clin. Endocrinol. Metab.* **46**, 816–823.

van Paassen, H. C., Poortman, J., Borgart-Creutzburg, I. H. C., Thijssen, J. H. H. and Duursma, S. A. (1978). Oestrogen binding proteins in bone cell cytosol. *Calcif. Tissue Res.* **25**, 249–254.

van Thiel, D. H. and Lester, R. (1976). Alcoholism: Its effect on hypothalamic pituitary gonadal function. *Gastroenterology* **71**, 318–327.

van Thiel, D. H., Gavaler, J. S., Lester, R. and Sherins, R. J. (1978). Alcohol-induced ovarian failure in the rat. *J. Clin. Invest.* **61**, 624–632.

van Wagenen, G. (1972). Vital statistics from a breeding colony: Reproduction and pregnancy outcome in *Macaca mulatta. J. Med. Primatol.* **1**, 3–28.

Vasquez, A. M. and Kenny, F. M. (1973). Ovarian failure and antiovarian antibodies in association with hypoparathyroidism, moniliasis, and Addison's and Hashimoto's Diseases. *Obstet. Gynecol.* **41**, 414–418.

Vekemans, M. and Robyn, C. (1975). Influence of age on serum prolactin levels in women and men. *Br. Med. J.* **4**, 738–739.

Vermeulen, A. (1976). The hormonal activity of the postmenopausal ovary. *J. Clin. Endocrinol. Metab.* **42**, 247–253.

Vermeulen, A. (1980). Sex hormone status of the postmenopausal woman. *Maturitas* **2**, 81–89.

Vermuelen, A. and Verdonck, L. (1978). Sex hormone concentrations in post-menopausal women. Relation to obesity, fat mass and years post-menopause. *Clin. Endocrinol. (Oxford)* **9**, 59–66.

Vermeulen, A., Deslypere, J. P., Schelfhout, W., Verdonck, L. and Rubens, R. (1982). Adrenocortical function in old age: Response to acute adrenocorticotropin stimulation. *J. Clin. Endocrinol. Metab.* **54**, 187–191.

Vessey, M. P., McPherson, K. and Johnson, B. (1977). Mortality among women participating in the Oxford/Family Planning Association contraceptive study. *Lancet* **2**, 731–733.

Vessey, M. P., Lawless, M., McPherson, K. and Yeates, D. (1983). Neoplasia of the cervix uteri and contraception: A possible adverse effect of the pill. *Lancet* **2**, 930–934.

Villanueva, A. L. and Rebar, R. W. (1983). Triple-X syndrome and premature ovarian failure. *Obset. Gynecol.* **62**, Suppl., 70S–73S.

Vittek, J., Altman, K., Gordon, G. C. and Southren, A. L. (1974). The metabolism of 7α-^{3}H-testosterone by rat mandibular bone. *Endocrinology* **94**, 325–329.

Vollman, R. F. (1977). The menstrual cycle. *In* "Major Problems in Obstetrics and Gynecology" (E. A. Friedman, ed.), Vol. 7, pp. 19–188. Saunders, Philadelphia, Pennsylvania.

Wajsbort, J. (1972). Post-menopausal bleeding after L-DOPA. *N. Engl. J. Med.* **286**, 784.

Waldeyer, W. (1870). "Eierstock und Ei." Engelmann, Leipzig.

Wallace, R. B., Sherman, B. M., Bean, J. A., Leeper, J. P. and Treloar, A. E. (1978). Menstrual cycle patterns and breast cancer risk factors. *Cancer Res.* **38**, 4021–4024.

Wallace, R. B., Sherman, B. M., Bean, J. A., Treloar, A. E. and Schlabaugh, L. (1979). Probability of menopause with increasing duration of amenorrhea in middle-aged women. *Am. J. Obstet. Gynecol.* **135**, 1021–1024.

Walsh, J. (1978). The age of the menopause of Australian women. *Med. J. Aust.* **2**, 181–215.

Wang, C., Hsueh, A. J. W. and Erickson, G. F. (1982). The role of cyclic AMP in the induction of estrogen and progestin synthesis in cultured granulosa cells. *Mol. Cell. Endocrinol.* **25**, 73–83.

Warburton, D., Stein, Z. and Kline, J. (1983). In utero selection against fetuses with trisomy. *Am. J. Hum. Genet.* **35**, 1059–1064.

Ware, H. (1979). Social influences on fertility at later ages of reproduction. *J. Biosocial Sci., Suppl.* **6**, 75–96.

Warne, G. L., Fairley, K. F., Hobbs, J. B. and Martin, F. I. R. (1973). Cyclophosphamide-induced ovarian failure. *N. Engl. J. Med.* **289**, 1159–1162.

Weinstein, G. D., Frost, P. and Hsia, S. L. (1968). *In vitro* interconversion of estrone and 17β-estradiol in human skin and vaginal mucosa. *J. Invest. Dermatol.* **51**, 4–10.

Weismann, A. (1885). "Die continuität des Keimplasmas als Grundlage einer Theorie der Verer-bung." Jena (cited from Hegner, 1914).

Weiss, N. C., Ure, C. L., Ballard, J. H., Williams, A. R. and Daling, J. R. (1980). Decreased risk of fractures of the hip and lower forearm with postmenopausal use of estrogen. *N. Engl. J. Med.* **303**, 1195–1198.

West, C. D., Damast, B. L., Sarro, S. D. and Pearson, O. H. (1956). Conversion of testosterone to estrogens in castrated, adrenalectomized human females. *J. Biol. Chem.* **218**, 409–418.

Wexler, B. C. (1964). Spontaneous arteriosclerosis in repeatedly bred male and female rats. *J. Atheroscler. Res.* **4**, 57–80.

Wide, L. (1981). Electrophoretic and gel chromatographic analyses of follicle-stimulating hormone in human serum. *Upsala J. Med. Sci.* **86**, 249–258.

Wide, L. (1982). Male and female forms of human follicle stimulating hormone in serum. *J. Clin. Endocrinol. Metab.* **55**, 682–688.

Wide, L. and Hobson, B. M. (1983). Qualitative difference in follicle-stimulating hormone activity in the pituitaries of young women compared to that of men and elderly women. *J. Clin. Endocrinol. Metab.* **56**, 371–375.

Wide, L. and Wide, M. (1984). Higher plasma disappearance rate in the mouse for pituitary follicle-stimulating hormone of young women compared to that of men and elderly women. *J. Clin. Endocrinol. Metab.* **58**, 426–429.

Wide, L., Nillius, S. J., Gemzell, C. and Roos, P. (1973). Radioimmunosorbent assay of follicle-stimulating hormone and luteinizing hormone in serum and urine from men and women. *Acta Endocrinol. (Copenhagen), Suppl.* **174**, 1–58.

Wigglesworth, J. S. (1964). Experimental growth retardation in the foetal rat. *J. Pathol. Bacteriol.* **88**, 1–13.

Wilbush, J. (1979). La ménespausie—the birth of a syndrome. *Maturitas* **1**, 145–151.

Wildt, L., Marshall, G. and Knobil, E. (1980). Experimental induction of puberty in the infantile female rhesus monkey. *Science* **207**, 1373–1375.

Wildt, L., Häusler, A., Hutchison, J. S., Marshall, G. and Knobil, E. (1981a). Estradiol as a gonadotropin releasing hormone in the rhesus monkey. *Endocrinology* **108**, 2011–2013.

Wildt, L., Häusler, A., Marshall, G., Hutchison, J. S., Plant, T. M., Belchetz, P. E. and Knobil, E. (1981b). Frequency and amplitude of gonadotropin-releasing hormone stimulation and gonadotropin secretion in the rhesus monkey. *Endocrinology* **109**, 376–385.

Williams, J. B. and Sharp, P. J. (1978). Age-dependent changes in the hypothalamo-pituitary-ovarian axis of the laying hen. *J. Reprod. Fertil.* **53**, 141–146.

Wise, P. M. (1982a). Alterations in proestrous LH, FSH and prolactin surges in middle-aged rats. *Proc. Soc. Exp. Biol. Med.* **169**, 348–354.

Wise, P. M. (1982b). Norepinephrine and dopamine activity in microdissected brain areas of the middle-aged and young rat on proestrus. *Biol. Reprod.* **27**, 562–574.

Wise, P. M. and Camp, P. (1984). Changes in concentrations of estradiol nuclear receptors in the preoptic area, medial basal hypothalamus, amygdala, and pituitary gland of middle-aged and old cycling rats. *Endocrinology* **114**, 92–98.

Witschi, E. (1948). Migration of the germ cells of human embryos from the yolk sac to the primitive gonadal folds. *Contrib. Embryol. Carnegie Inst.* **32**, 67–80.

Witt, M. F. and Blethen, S. L. (1983). The endocrine evaluation of three children with vasomotor flushes following hypothalamic surgery. *Clin. Endocrinol. (Oxford)* **18**, 551–555.

Woessner, J. F., Jr. (1963). Age related changes of the human uterus and its connective tissue framework. *J. Gerontol.* **18**, 220–226.

World Health Organization (1981). "Research on the Menopause," W. H. O. Tech. Rep. Ser. No. 670. WHO, Geneva.

Wyon, J. B., Finner, S. L. and Gordon, J. E. (1966). Differential age at menopause in the rural Punjab, India. *Popul. Index* **32**, 328.

Yen, S. S. C. (1980). The polycystic ovary syndrome. *Clin. Endocrinol. (Oxford)* **12**, 177–208.

Yen, S. S. C. (1983). Clinical applications of gonadotropin-releasing hormone and gonadotropin-releasing hormone analogs. *Fertil. Steril.* **39**, 257–266.

Young, M. M. and Nordin, B. E. C. (1967). Effects of natural and artificial menopause on plasma and urinary calcium and phosphorus. *Lancet* **2**, 118–120.

YoungLai, E. V. and Short, R. V. (1970). Pathways of steroid biosynthesis in the intact Graafian follicle of mares in oestrus. *J. Endocrinol.* **47**, 321–331.

Zander, J., Brendle, E., von Münstermann, A.-M., Diczfalusy, E., Martinsen, B. and Tillinger, K.-G. (1959). Identification and estimation of estradiol-17β and oestrone in human ovaries. *Acta Obstet. Gynecol. Scand.* **38**, 724–736.

Zelesnik, A. J., Schuler, H. M. and Reichert, L. E., Jr. (1981). Gonadotropin-binding sites in the rhesus monkey ovary: Role of the vasculature in the selective distribution of human chorionic gonadotropin to the preovulatory follicle. *Endocrinology* **109**, 356–362.

Zoller, L. C. and Weisz, J. (1978). Identification of cytochrome P-450, and its distribution in the membrana granulosa of the preovulatory follicle, using quantitative cytochemistry. *Endocrinology* **103**, 310–313.

Zumoff, B., Rosenfeld, R. S., Strain, G. W., Levin, J. and Fukushima, D. K. (1980). Sex differences in the twenty-four-hour mean plasma concentrations of dehydroisoandrosterone (DHA) and dehydroisoandrosterone sulfate (DHAS) and the DHA to DHAS ratio in normal adults. *J. Clin. Endocrinol. Metab.* **51**, 330–333.

Index

Date Due

JAN 3 1 1990			
3 1 1990			
JAN 3 1 1990			

BRODART, INC.　　　　Cat. No. 23 233　　　　Printed in U.S.A.